THE SANCTITY
OF HUMAN LIFE

THE SANCTITY
OF HUMAN LIFE

~

David Novak

GEORGETOWN UNIVERSITY PRESS
Washington, D.C.

As of January 1, 2007, 13-digit ISBN numbers
have replaced the 10-digit system.

13-digit   10-digit
Cloth: 978-1-58901-176-2   Cloth: 1-58901-176-7

Georgetown University Press, Washington, D.C.
www.press.georgetown.edu

Library of Congress Cataloging-in-Publication Data
Novak, David, 1941–
The sanctity of human life / David Novak.
p. ; cm.
Includes bibliographical references and index.
ISBN-13: 978-1-58901-176-2 (cloth : alk. paper)
ISBN-10: 1-58901-176-7 (cloth : alk. paper)
1. Medical ethics—Religious aspects—Judaism. 2. Embryonic stem
cells—Research—Religious aspects—Judaism. 3. Social medicine—
Religious aspects—Judaism. 4. Assisted suicide—Religious aspects—
Judaism. I. Title.
[DNLM: 1. Judaism. 2. Philosophy, Medical. 3. Ethics, Medical. 4.
Life. 5. Religion and Medicine. W 61 N934 2007]
R725.57.N68 2007
174.2—dc22
2007007013

∞ This book is printed on acid-free paper meeting the requirements
of the American National Standard for Permanence in Paper
for Printed Library Materials.

14 13 12 11 10 09 08 07   9 8 7 6 5 4 3 2
First printing
Printed in the United States of America

To
Batsheva Chaya Stadlan
Hillel Hadar Stadlan
Jordan Ahava Novak

"Children of children are like one's own children."
(BABYLONIAN TALMUD: YEVAMOT 62B)

CONTENTS

PREFACE

The term "the sanctity of human life" has a definite religious ring. It seems to denote the fact that human life is related to God. Moreover, although the term "sanctity of human life" (*qedushat ha-hayyim*) does not appear—to my knowledge—in any of the classical Jewish sources, all the classical Jewish discussions of the life-and-death questions with which I deal in the three essays here certainly assume the idea. Does that mean this term can only be used in theological discussions of the normative issues to which this term and the idea it names pertains? If that is the case, how can the idea of the sanctity of human life enter philosophical and political discussions in which not all discussants hold theological assumptions about God and humans' relationship with God? Clearly, in the secular space in which basic questions of public philosophy and policy are discussed today, one cannot assume any theological consensus, even among worshipers of the same God, even in the same faith—let alone among those in different faith communities. So how can one use a theologically charged idea such as the sanctity of human life in the absence of any general theological consensus anywhere?

This question leaves a Jewish theologian such as myself, who is very much concerned with the normative issues I discuss in this book as they are raised both within my tradition and within the world at large, with a dilemma. I could confine my discussion of the sanctity of human life to theological reflection on how it operates within the normative Jewish tradition—that is, the way it has operated in decisions already made and the way it ought to operate in decisions now to be made. I would have to find a more secular idea, however, when I speak as an ethicist or moral philosopher in a secular context. After all, the normative questions I discuss here—stem-cell research, universal health care, and physician-assisted suicide—arise in universities, research laboratories, government bureaus, and hospitals, not in synagogues, yeshivahs, or rabbinical courts (and not in churches, theological seminaries, or ecclesiastical courts either, lest it be thought my problem is only a Jewish one). Therefore, I try to show that the theological meaning of the sanctity of human life in the context of the God–human relationship is itself related to the idea of the sanctity of human life in the context of interhuman relationships with which philosophical ethics certainly is concerned. I can do so while working within the Jewish tradition because there is no issue in the God–human relationship that does not have a correlate in the interhuman relationship, and vice versa. Yet I must interrelate theology and philosophy to contend with these three normative questions (or any normative questions) in a way that does not derive philosophy from theology or theology from philosophy, or politics from either of them—something that would ruin all three areas of public discourse and action.

One can see this connection between the theological meaning of the sanctity of human life and the philosophical meaning of that term when one distinguishes between theology and philosophy as follows: Theology deals with the God–human relationship primarily and interhuman relationships secondarily; philosophy, especially as ethics, deals with interhuman relationships primarily and maximally can allude to the God–human relationship when it accepts, minimally, the possibility of that relationship in the world. Politics adopts both theological and philosophical uses of the sanctity of human life.

To make this point clearer, consider the use of the Hebrew term for "sacred" or "holy"—*qadosh*—first in its original context and then in terms of how it pertains to human life by analogy. (Some of the sources on which I draw in making this analogy are II Kings 12:2; Ezekiel 42:20, 48:15; *Mishnah*, Meilah 3.6 [and Maimonides, *Commentary on the Mishnah* thereon], 5.1; *Tosefta*, Meilah 1.21, 23; Maimonides, *Mishneh Torah:* Meilah, 8.1; and *Mishnah*, Yoma 1.3.) In the original scriptural sources, *qadosh* denotes the separation of something from its ordinary use in the world for the sake of what lies beyond the world. Most specifically and most often in Scripture, *qadosh* pertains to entities—humans or animals or things (*qodashim*)—that are "holy unto the Lord" (Leviticus 27:32). This separation has two meanings: one positive, the other negative.

The positive meaning of *qadosh* pertains to how these sacred entities function as Temple offerings to please God or as articles these offerings require for their proper preparation as offerings that are pleasing to God. Thus, they are positively used by the persons who are charged with preparing them and offering them up to God. Only those who are personally involved in these ministrations can possibly experience the sacred relationship positively, however, and thus understand its essential meaning within the confines of the Temple itself. In other words, that experience and the understanding of its meaning can come only from the relationship these Temple ministers have with God, into which these sacred things have become the means thereto.

The negative meaning of *qadosh* pertains to how persons outside the ministrations of the Temple are related to those sacred things. For them, these sacred things are only inviolable. That is, they are neither to be harmed in any way nor used for any worldly purpose. Even worldly use that does not harm these sacred things removes them from their separation from or transcendence of the world by making them a commodity of one sort or another. In fact, even outsiders employed to do work for the Temple—without whose work the Temple could not be built, be maintained, or function—are not to be paid from the sacred things themselves but from other funds, so that the transcendence of the sacred things themselves is not compromised. Furthermore, even if these outsiders (*zarim*) may have heard of how the sacred things function in the Temple, they must respectfully refrain from violating them. Because these sacred things are not part of these outsiders' own personal experience, however, they cannot very well understand what all this truly means. As such, they cannot speak about what has no meaning outside the Temple. As Wittgenstein aptly notes, "Of that which we cannot speak, about that we must be silent" (*Tractatus Logico-Politicus*, 7). This is not to suggest, however, that we deny the reality of what we cannot speak by our silence about it in foreign contexts.

For the ministers of the Temple, who have a positive experience of the Temple rites and what they intend, the negative can be derived from the positive. That is, because these sacred things play such an important role in the full cosmic scheme of creation, they should not be harmed or used for anything other than their essential function. Yet even persons who are outside this sacred circle can understand the negative significance of these sacred things, even if such outsiders cannot infer the negative from the positive. They can reach this understanding from their own experience—which is that these things have always been protected from any violation or exploitation because they seem to reflect something beyond themselves, even if they cannot say what that "something beyond" really is. Hence, even though they cannot derive the negative—this sense of respectful restraint—from anything positive in their own experience, they can sense enough of an allusion to "something beyond" that they would not reduce these sacred things to their own worldly use or misuse. For them the sacred is mysterious.

Thus, although the ministers of the Temple and outsiders can come to the same practical conclusion regarding nonworldly use of sacred things, they cannot and should not use each other's logic in coming to that conclusion. They can only appreciate that use of one logic in one context does not rule out use of another logic in another context, even when the discourses structured by these respective logics are talking about the same thing.

The analogue to this dichotomy regarding sacred things in the question of the sanctity of human life is as follows: Religious people experience the sanctity of human life in their own lives when they are positively related to God. Jews call that relationship a "covenant" (*berit*); the constitution of this relationship is the Torah, and it is acted out by the performance of the commandments (*mitsvot*). Realizing that what they experience is a possibility for any human being, they infer that all human life is inviolable and is not to be exploited in any way because of that possibility, whether it is realized or not. These religious people are like the people who minister within the precincts of the Temple and have tasted the intensity of what obtains there. They know that the sanctuary and its sacred things must not be violated or exploited by anyone—that such violation would contradict the reality they have so intensely experienced and in which they have so actively participated.

Nonreligious people (or religious people whose relationship with God has no significance for their morally charged relations in the secular realm) cannot be expected to draw any such inference because they have no positive basis from which to draw it. Nevertheless, they can appreciate that human life alludes to more than

merely being a thing in the world that can be destroyed or exploited. This appreciation often comes out of their experience of
injustice. That is, they cannot accept the reduction of human beings to the status of mere things, which is what injustice assumes.
Even though they cannot or will not offer any positive reasons that
are otherworldly to counter the reductive assumption underlying
all injustice and what is invoked to rationalize it, they refuse to be
persuaded by these rationalizations. Their experience of injustice
has taught them that when these mundane assumptions about the
ordinariness of human life are put into practice, the result is the
degradation of human life to a point of disgust of every human life,
including their own. Human life on these terms is not worth living.
These nonreligious people are like the people outside the Temple
who have not experienced what goes on there yet do not want to
violate or exploit what seems to reflect a reality that is beyond what
can ever be violated or exploited in the world. Moreover, just as
theologians (*hakhamim*) should instruct persons who participate in
the life of the Temple how and why they are to treat the sacred
things in a way God deserves because of who God is, the philosophers (who also are *hakhamim*) should instruct persons outside the
Temple how and why to treat human beings in a way they deserve
because of who they are.

Following the analogy to holy things, people who can only pos-
tulate rather than constitute the sanctity of human life are like the
people outside the Temple who have never experienced, let alone
handled, the holy things, yet can still appreciate that (if not yet
why) they are not to be violated or used for any mundane purpose.
In that way, the priests (*kohanim*) in the Temple could communi-
cate to outsiders (*zarim*) a message about the inviolability of the
holy things, even though they cannot impose upon these outsiders
their understanding of the positive meaning of these holy things.
After all, these outsiders have never experienced, let alone handled,
what lies within the Temple. There can be no understanding without experience of and with what is to be understood.

Finally, all the theologians need from the philosophers is that the
philosophers not deny the possibility of the revelation from which
the theologians receive their basic norms. All the philosophers need
from the theologians is that the theologians not argue from the

authority of revelation and its tradition when they are speaking outside the sacred precincts of their Temple. When both sides accept those preconditions, a conversation about the sanctity of human life is possible at the border between theology and philosophy—a conversation in which the very term "sanctity" can have multiple yet not mutually exclusive meanings.

That is why I have titled the book comprising these three essays *The Sanctity of Human Life*. I hope readers will see that idea as the unifying feature of these three chapters and agree that this term can be cogently used in theological, philosophical, and political contexts. Moreover, as in my previous books, there is a text and a subtext. In the text I have tried to present arguments that are meant to be intelligible (perhaps even persuasive) to readers of general backgrounds and interests. In the longer notes, however, I try to show how my arguments have been developed out of a wide variety of textual resources. In fact, I hope that readers with more specialized interests (in Judaism or secular bodies of knowledge) will look up some of the sources I cite and discuss in the notes to check how responsible I have been in my use of these sources, in addition to how accurate my citation of them has been.

The breakdown of the chapters into their various subsections, as shown in the table of contents, indicates the subtopics of each of the chapters and how they are ordered. That breakdown is a better initial indication of what I am saying than a too-brief summary of each chapter of the kind one often finds in prefaces of collections of essays. Therefore, I simply offer a little background to each of the three essays.

The first chapter, "On the Use of Embryonic Stem Cells," began in a paper I delivered at Fordham University Law School in May 2002. I am grateful for comments by persons who were present for that talk, especially the comments of Professor Suzanne Last Stone of Cardozo Law School of Yeshiva University, who was the official respondent to my paper. I also benefited from conversations with my friend and colleague, Professor Robert George of Princeton University, who also is the director of the James Madison Program in American Ideals and Institutions there, of whose Board of Consulting Scholars I am proud to be a founding member. During the spring semester of 2006, when I was a visiting professor of religion and a William E. Simon Fellow at Princeton, Professor George and I were able to regularly discuss some of the great moral issues involved in embryonic stem cell research. He helpfully shared with me his experiences as a member of the commission charged by the President of the United States with dealing with this question.

The second chapter, "A Jewish Argument for Socialized Medicine," began as the Isaac Franck Memorial Lecture at the Kennedy Institute of Ethics at Georgetown University in June 2003. (I was especially honored to deliver this lecture in memory of Dr. Isaac Franck, a philosopher who served as the executive director of the Jewish Federation of Greater Washington in the 1960s, who befriended and guided me as a young rabbi and graduate student in philosophy during that turbulent time.) This essay was subsequently published, with minor changes, under the same title in the *Kennedy Institute of Ethics Journal* 13 (2003): 313–28. Because of this article, Dr. Richard Brown, director of Georgetown University Press, invited me to write this book for the press. I happily accepted his kind invitation. It was a special privilege to be so invited by the distinguished press of Georgetown University, which conferred my Ph.D. in philosophy in May 1971. As a Georgetown alumnus, I very much appreciate the help of the editorial staff in getting my manuscript through the publication process so skillfully.

The third chapter, on "Physician-Assisted Suicide," began as a graduate course on that topic that I taught at the University of Toronto in the spring semester of 1998. I learned a great deal from the students in that course—especially Dr. Michael Gordon, medical director of the Baycrest Geriatric Centre in Toronto, who took the course while he was a student in the Joint Centre for Bioethics of the university (of which I am a faculty member). More recently, I delivered the Krovonsha Lecture in Bioethics at Loma Linda University in California on this topic. I am grateful to the attentive and inquisitive audience that attended that lecture. Thanks also are due to Dr. Mark Carr, now of the faculty of Loma Linda University, who was my student at the University of Virginia in the early 1990s and invited me to deliver this lecture. Most recently, I delivered the Dr. Saul Green Memorial Lecture on this topic at the Faculty of Medicine of Dalhousie University in Halifax, Nova Scotia. There too, I learned much from an attentive and inquisitive audience.

I have discussed many of the classical Jewish texts represented and interpreted in this book with my friend, Rabbi Arnold Turin of Toronto. As always, I have benefited enormously from his learning and his wisdom (whether we agreed or agreed not to agree on the meaning of what we have discussed together). I also thank my University of Toronto colleague Timothy Barnes for helping me locate the classical Greek sources of the modern term "euthanasia."

Once again, Matthew LaGrone, my Ph.D. student and research assistant at the University of Toronto, deserves grateful mention. He was especially helpful in locating important contemporary literature (in print and on the Internet) that was pertinent to the main topics of this book. He also offered much good editorial advice and carefully prepared the index. I want to thank David Stearman for his superb job of editing, especially some of the philosophical questions he raised that helped me refine my argument when I was rewriting some key passages in the body of the text of this book.

Finally, the dedication: When my first grandchild—Zehavya Stadlan, the firstborn child of my children Marianne Novak and Dr. Noam Y. Stadlan—was born, I was very proud to dedicate my book *Natural Law in Judaism* (Cambridge University Press, 1998) to her. Now, thank God, there are three more grandchildren: Marianne and Noam's daughter Batsheva (born in 1998) and son Hillel (born in 2001) and Jordan (born in 2003), the daughter of our children Jacob and Adar Novak. I am now proud to dedicate this book to these three grandchildren, whose parents are raising them to respect the sanctity of all human life in word and in deed. That legacy makes my wife and me proud of them and their parents. This dedication is my way of telling others how my wife and I feel about them (see Zohar 1:233a regarding Genesis 48:20). We truly live and work for those whom we love.

1

ON THE USE OF EMBRYONIC
STEM CELLS

NORMATIVE QUESTIONS AND NORMATIVE CONTEXTS

The current moral debate about the use of embryonic stem cells for the possible (some advocates might even say probable) saving of other human lives is so intense because—as of 2007—deriving "pluripotent" (useful) stem cells from embryos kills these embryos in the process. This debate takes place in several different contexts: scientific, philosophical, political, and theological. Although complete discussion of an issue such as stem cell research must take all four of these contexts into consideration, one should specify the particular context of any such discussion.

Because we are dealing with a moral question that arises out of new scientific research on prenatal life, we should begin our discussion in that context—even though we are approaching this context of the discussion with our ethical commitments already in hand. Hence, ethicists on one side of the debate regarding stem cell research use the scientific differentiation of the stages of prenatal life to bolster their moral differentiation of the stages of prenatal life by attempting to show that their moral differentiation is not arbitrary but has some basis in scientifically established fact. Conversely, ethicists on the other side of the debate deny that this scientific differentiation of the stages of prenatal life has any moral significance and that prenatal life at any stage of its development deserves protection from harm or extinction. Whereas the first group of ethicists uses the specific differences in the stages of prenatal life to bolster their moral argument, the second group of ethicists uses the genetic commonality of all prenatal life to bolster their moral argument. Thus, both sides use scientific evidence to escape charges of arbitrariness in dealing with a moral issue that itself arises out of scientific research. Nevertheless, although science lends itself to moral reasoning, especially in issues that affect its practice, it does not decide what one ought to do with the data and interpretations of data it has provided. Questions of what one ought to do are properly discussed in philosophical, theological, and political contexts.

Scientists distinguish between a zygote or preembryo (an egg fertilized by a sperm but not yet implanted into the uterine wall, which usually occurs within ten to fourteen days after fertilization), an embryo (an egg fertilized by a sperm that has been implanted into the uterine wall), and a fetus (an implanted embryo after about the eighth week of gestation). Because pluripotent stem cells are derived from preembryos that have been kept in a petri dish rather than having been implanted into the uterine wall (as intended in vitro fertilization), in the interest of scientific accuracy one should speak of stem cells being derived from preembryos. To be more precise: Such cells come from young embryos, termed blastocysts, that are only a few days old.[1]

Some ethicists—Jewish and non-Jewish alike—use this scientific differentiation to assert a moral difference between a zygote and an embryo, arguing that one may treat a preembryo differently from the way one may treat an embryo. Other ethicists argue that there is no such moral difference (although there is a theological difference in certain cases), just as there is no moral difference between the way one may treat an embryo and the way one may treat a fetus. The commonality in kind between a zygote and an embryo—namely, that they both possess the same unique DNA—outweighs any differences in degree between their respective stages of prenatal development. Counting myself among the latter group of ethicists, I use the term "embryo" consistently in discussing stem cell research, for moral reasons and for greater terminological simplicity. I reserve use of the term "fetus" in addressing the issue of abortion in the usual sense—namely, extraction of a fetus already in utero. Embryos that are used for stem cell research, however, are conceived through in vitro fertilization, which is an extrauterine procedure.

For both sides in this intense debate over stem cell research using live embryos, the issue is a matter of life and death. The debate involves three distinct moral questions: May stem cells be derived from live embryos? Should stem cells be derived from live embryos? Should stem cells not be derived from live embryos?

What *may* be done is an option that can be done with impunity. The act is permitted insofar as an applicable norm (legal, moral, or religious) does not prohibit the act from being done, although there is no obligation for anyone to actually do it. One cannot infer that something *should* be done from mere permission that it *may* be done (even though what may be done eventually can become a low-level obligation either by statute or by custom).[2] What *should not* be done and what *may not* be done have identical normative meanings, however, inasmuch as they both denote a negative obligation: a "thou shalt not."[3] Somebody who does what should not be done is a criminal when the transgressed norm is legal, a reprobate when the transgressed norm is moral, and a sinner when the transgressed norm is religious. Hence, whether we are speaking in a legal, moral, or religious context, we must ask whether derivation of stem cells from live embryos is permitted, obligated, or prohibited. In other words, is it optional, mandatory, or forbidden?

There are three contexts for the discussion of this question: political, philosophical, and theological. Any public discussion of this question that does not take all three contexts into consideration, separately and in correlation with each other, is myopic. Furthermore, the three contexts of this question (and others of similar social significance) inevitably overlap inasmuch as a Jewish thinker such as myself has a theological stake in the Jewish tradition, which can be shown to have philosophical significance on universal philosophical issues and can be applied in turn to political issues in the particular secular society in which I live. Therefore, before I can deal adequately with the actual normative question regarding the use of stem cells from live embryos and the three aforementioned formal normative questions, I must deal with the three contextual questions at some length. Moreover, this contextual discussion must take place along with the discussion of the normative question. Hence, this contextual discussion of politics, philosophy, and theology is interspersed throughout the normative discussion of the question regarding the use of stem cells from live embryos. Indeed, politics, philosophy, and theology are inherently normative disciplines.

By ignoring the need to contextualize the normative discussion, too many discussions of the issue of stem cell research and similar issues in bioethics have made very little impact because the persons to whom they are addressed can say all too frequently, "You are not talking *to* us; you are only taking *at* us. We do not recognize ourselves to be the persons to whom you are making your moral claims." In other words, practical moral claims can be made cogently to persons for their response only when the claimant and the respondent share a common normative domain.

Normative claims made by theologians are especially vulnerable to the charge of moral irrelevancy. Jewish theologians, especially, often fall into a pattern of simply declaring "the Jewish point of view" on some issue or other, without considering why anyone should act according to what Jewish theologians represent to be a Jewish norm. Thus, when a Jewish norm is addressed to a non-Jewish audience, that audience can easily reject it by saying (or simply thinking), "But we are not Jews, nor do we intend to convert to Judaism." Hence, a broader contextualization of the discussion is needed to better persuade individuals outside the tradition in which a particular theology has evolved that its discussion of an issue such as stem cell research does concern individuals who do not belong to that tradition—or, for that matter, even persons who do not belong to any tradition (or any tradition of which they are aware or admit). That broader contextualization must move into philosophy. It requires theologians to refine their moral reasoning, especially when they are required to speak philosophically to philosophers or even to their fellow citizens who want to hear philosophical arguments regarding issues of public policy such as the issue of stem cell research. In other words, in arguing for a particular normative conclusion—which surely is required of anyone who enters the stem cell debate—a Jewish theologian such as myself must show that his or her normative conclusion is true and not just Jewishly correct. Therefore, the discussion here is primarily philosophical, although I hope it will be consistent with the theological tradition of rabbinic Judaism. Moreover, the discussion is not oblivious to what might or might not be prudent politics in dealing with this and similar issues that arise in the public square.

Discussions that reduce this question or any question like it to the realm of politics or legal technicalities alone ignore the moral and philosophical questions of why anyone should obey the law of any polity or why anyone should morally advocate any new public policies. Reduction of normative questions to the realm of politics alone also ignores the fact that for most people in our society, morality is inexplicably bound up with their theology or religious outlook. That is so whether people are formally religious (in the sense that they are part of a religious or faith community), informally religious (an individualist metaphysical mindset that some people call spirituality), or even antireligious. One might say that almost all serious people have metaphysical commitments, whether they are formally religious or not.

One's outlook is metaphysical when it regards human nature (that is, one's humanity or essential humanness) as more than the mere sum of an individual's body parts and more than even the collective body politic. (*Meta* is a Greek prefix that can mean "beyond.") Once we get into what is beyond or transcendent, we cannot avoid the question of God, whether our answer is pro or con—which Nietzsche saw better than any other philosopher.[4] Thus, atheists—who think that to affirm human nature is to deny God—are no less metaphysical than theists who think that to affirm human nature is thereby to affirm the human relationship with God to be its very essence.[5] Metaphysical anthropology refuses to be dismissed as a pseudo-question. We must go beyond what most modern English-speaking philosophers, let alone most modern politicians anywhere, have taken to be of any importance. From here we need to connect metaphysics to ethics.

Metaphysical anthropology deals with what a human being *is;* ethics deals with what a human being *ought to do.* How are they connected? To recognize whether an act is intentionally human (that is, meant to be humanly done) or not, we must be able to recognize whether the actor is acting in an appropriately human way or not: in a way that is worthy or unworthy of a human person as a metaphysical being—a being whose very presence in the world points to what is beyond the world. That is what the essential sanctity or inviolability or dignity of human life means.[6] So, is the choice to do or not to do a particular act truly consistent with the sacred, inviolable, dignified human nature of the subject of the act, or not? Is one acting like a human being or like a predatory animal? Given that ethics governs interpersonal transactions, is the act to be chosen or resisted consistent with the human nature of the object of the act or not? Am I respecting the other person before me for his or her human sanctity, inviolability, and dignity, or not? Am I treating the other person before me like a predatory animal toward whom violence is the only appropriate response? In other words, I am to act because of what I am, and I am to treat others because of what they are. In the case of my interpersonal transactions, my own actions and my actions toward whom or with whom I am acting are justified by the exact same reason. That fact alone distinguishes intelligent human action from unintelligent behavior—that is, whether that consciously willed action is justifiable in terms of its consistency with human nature. The human nature of both the moral subject and the moral object are expressed in the claims they make on each other and the choices they themselves make in the name of what they are and what they need. Human nature, then, is the true measure of human action.

The twentieth-century Jewish philosopher Martin Buber showed that human nature is essentially relational, and its essential relationships are all externally constituted.[7] Even internal relations within the mind (what some philosophers like to call "inner experience") are either traces of external relationships from the past or anticipations of external relationships yet to be. That relational aspect is at the core of human nature and has ethical implications for those of us who bear that human nature as its acting subjects and acted-upon objects. Indeed, no human subject of "I" acts in an ethical vacuum without intending another human object as a "thou," and every human object or "me" discovers his or her humanity when he or she is addressed by another person as a "thou."[8]

To act in a dignified human way and to treat other humans with equal dignity is to affirm the truth of human nature in practice. To act otherwise and to treat other humans otherwise is to lie, whether in word or deed. Human nature by its very presence prescribes, as it were, its own affirmation and proscribes its own denial by both the human subjects and the human objects who bear it because our human nature manifests itself primarily in the claims others make on us and the claims we make on others. Thus, the opposite of the practical affirmation of the truth of personhood is active lying or treachery, whereas the opposite of the theoretical affirmation of the truth of descriptive propositions is only error.[9] Unlike descriptive propositions, persons continually ask us to affirm in word and deed the truth of their personhood and our own personhood in our interpersonal transactions with them. Hence, persons ask us to act truthfully or faithfully *with* them in a way that descriptive propositions do not ask us to speak the truth *about* them. Affirming what is true of human nature entails an *ought:* an inherent obligation. Acting truthfully is being faithful to others and to ourselves along with them.

Moral objects are unlike the objects we encounter in our technological, scientific, and aesthetic experience of nature per se. In these kinds of impersonal experiences, as distinct from interpersonal transactions, all claims are made by us on the objects before us. Unlike personal objects, these impersonal objects do not seem to make any *prima facie* claims on us (with the possible exception of higher animals—a point to which I return later). Thus, we claim objects as useful for us technologically, intelligible scientifically, and beautiful or enjoyable aesthetically. Only with objects made by persons, such as *oeuvres d'art*, do the persons who made these objects make claims on us through them; that is, these artificial objects bespeak a message from their makers for us in one way or another. (Like any property, moreover, these artificial objects bespeak the claim of their owners that I do not harm them or steal them.) Therefore, a metaphysics of human nature, with its implications for human action, must be constituted in a fundamentally different way than a metaphysics of nature per se. (In a metaphysics of creation coming out of revelation, the commandment of God tells us who created and governs the nature we experience and how we are to act toward it. That commandment, however, does not come from our experience of nature without this theological mediation.)[10] In addition, whereas a philosophy of nature per se might be able to avoid the God question, a metaphysics of human nature cannot. If a metaphysics of human nature affirms God, it thereby affirms that human personhood (comprising intelligence, freedom, and efficacy) is transcended by One who has greater intelligence, freedom, and efficacy. If a metaphysics of human nature denies God, however, it thereby affirms that human intelligence, freedom, and efficacy (as distinct from raw power) transcend everything else in the universe. In one way or another, an atheistic metaphysics substitutes man for God. Whether theistic or atheistic, however, no metaphysics of human nature or philosophical anthropology can avoid the question of transcendence.

Such metaphysical reflection is an integral feature of an ethics that distinguishes action from behavior. An authentic human ethics presupposes a metaphysics of human nature, which Kant saw better than any other philosopher when he asserted that the only possible metaphysics is a metaphysics that is needed for ethics to be truly rational rather than simply prudential (what Kant called *Metaphysik der Sitten*).[11] Hence, the ethical value of an act depends on how consistent it is with human nature, metaphysically conceived. Moreover, whereas Kant could eliminate the God question from his metaphysics (or antimetaphysics) of nature per se, he had to deal with that question of all questions in his metaphysical treatment of morality, although one certainly can challenge the theological adequacy of his invocation of God there.[12]

Nevertheless, we do not directly derive ethics from metaphysics. We do not have a metaphysical view of human nature and then put it into practice. We are already acting in a certain way: doing *this* but not doing *that*, consciously and willfully. When we reflect on why we are doing *this* but not *that*, we see retrospectively that we act this way because of the way we regard both our own nature and the nature of those with whom we interact—a nature that is freely affirmed or denied by the way we act. That reflection is what distinguishes intentional action from unintentional behavior. A metaphysically charged ethics, however, is not a theoretical premise waiting for us to draw a practical conclusion from it. In fact, if we did not have considerable ethical experience first, we would be in no position to understand why we do what we do—that is, what makes our ethical action truly intelligent (a point best made by Aristotle).[13] A metaphysics of ethics is a metaphysics for ethics, and it is constituted *post factum*.

Persons who do regard their morality as without metaphysical foundation—true agnostics—inevitably fall into the ethical dead-end of legalism, which is an irrational, absolute commitment to a system of secular, human-made, positive law. The question of whether that law is made by someone as benevolent as Gandhi or as malevolent as Hitler cannot make any real difference to these agnostics. In other words, they cannot give a metaphysically cogent reason for why they obey anyone. All they can say is that they obey whoever has political authority over them because they will be either punished for their disobedience or rewarded for their obedience. How does that attitude differ, however, from the motivation of a dog to obey its master?[14] As such, these agnostics have reduced ethics to power politics instead of regarding the political realm as the primary context for a person to act ethically according to his or her metaphysically constituted human nature.

Discussions that reduce a question such as the use of embryonic stem cells to philosophy alone thereby ignore the political question of what can or cannot be accomplished in any real society. Moreover, they cannot deal with the fact that even in today's world, morality and metaphysics—which for most serious people is their theology—go hand-in-hand. Conversely, discussions that reduce the question to theology seem to presume that we are living in a theocracy—which is not the case for most of the world, with the notable exceptions of states such as Saudi Arabia and Iran. Philosophy and politics are not to be deduced from theology any more than they are to be deduced from each other; they need only be correlated with theology for a truly comprehensive public policy in a secular yet multicultural society in which most people are religious, whether formally or informally, and almost everyone (except the type of bureaucrats for whom the political realm is their all-encompassing reality) has some sort of metaphysical commitment. That metaphysical commitment is either theological or antitheological.

Philosophy can only allude to a metaphysical dimension of human existence; it cannot constitute that dimension because metaphysics without God as its prime object of interest is uninteresting. Since Kant, moreover, philosophy has been unable to talk about God. When it attempts to do so, the God it conjures up bears little or no resemblance to the God the members of any living historical culture worship. The most philosophy can contribute to modern "God-talk" is to provide particular theologies that are still being formulated within living historical cultures with the tools for analysis of their own God-talk or for a phenomenology of the experiences of which that God-talk speaks.

Regardless, an adequate treatment of a question such as the use of stem cells derived from living embryos must take the interrelation of law, morality, and religion into account continually, even when the discussion takes place in only one of these contexts primarily. More precisely, this can be regarded as the relation of positive law, universal morality, and revelation. (There is a longstanding practice of calling universal morality natural law, so I use the two terms interchangeably.) The fact that law, morality, and religion are related does not mean that they are identical, however. Thus, there can be acts that are permitted because they are not explicitly prohibited legally, although they are not morally or religiously mandated or even morally or religiously permitted. Consider the legal status of adultery in our secular societies: It has long ceased to be a crime in the legal sense (and with the advent of "no fault" divorce in most western societies already, adultery cannot even be grounds for divorce because one no longer needs any grounds or reasons to divorce one's spouse). Moreover, there can be acts that are not legally mandated but can be morally or religiously permitted or even morally or religiously mandated. Giving charity, for example, falls in this category.

In the case at hand, there are two opposing moral proposals. At best, both proposals are philosophical. On one hand, advocates say that although use of stem cells derived from live embryos, which entails killing the embryos in the process, is not explicitly prohibited by the positive law of the state, it may not or should not be done for moral reasons, even if those stem cells might save other human lives. (Whether it could actually be prohibited legally is improbable because abortion on demand is permitted in almost every western society.) That one human life should not be taken to save another human life seems to be rationally evident. On the other hand, however, use of such stem cells possibly (or even probably) could save other human lives. In this view, because the status of the embryo, especially in the first week or so of its life, is doubtfully human and the lives its stem cells might save certainly are human, what is certain should trump what is doubtful.[15] In this view, we are not destroying one human life in favor of another equally human life (or lives).

The principle that one human life ought not be taken to save another human life applies only when the two lives are of equal worth or sanctity. For example, we would say in a case of self-defense, where the only way to save the life of the would-be victim is to kill the attacker, that the attacker has forfeited his or her right to life in favor of the right to life of his or her would-be victim because the only way to prevent the attacker's unjustified intent to kill from being exercised is to kill the attacker first. This example is the one notable exception to the norm that one life ought not be destroyed for the sake of another.[16] Moreover, most of us would not grant that exception when the attacker could be prevented from murdering a would-be victim by means other than killing that attacker.[17] Following this logic, some advocates of unlimited stem cell research have argued that the embryo from *which* (not from *whom*) the stem cell is to be derived has also forfeited its life in the interest of a greater good. In this view, minimally we *may* derive stem cells from living embryos whatever the consequences; maximally, we *should* do so. Usually, the maximal position is argued by proponents of stem cell research involving the killing of embryos.

Thus, there are two opposing moral proposals regarding the derivation of stem cells from live embryos that kills their donor in the process. That is, the only two cogent alternative answers to our question appear to be the following: Stem cells should not be derived from living embryos because their derivation kills these embryos, or stem cells should be derived from living embryos, even if these embryos are killed in the process, because these stem cells can save other lives that are more human than the embryos that had to be killed for their sake. These two proposals are mutually exclusive, and I see no way to effect a compromise between them. The only possible candidate for such a compromise would be to make taking stem cells from living embryos optional—that is, neither prohibited nor mandated. That option, however, apparently would satisfy neither side in the debate.

For people who want a prohibition of stem cell research involving living embryos, there is no real difference (only a logical distinction) between permitting something and mandating it. Doesn't public permission of an act such as euthanasia (which previously has been prohibited) imply that this act is what society wants? (Consider "voluntary" euthanasia in The Netherlands today.)

For advocates who want a mandate for stem cell research involving living embryos, mere permission is too weak to bring about what they want. Because people who argue for this second proposal want a governmental mandate (and funding) for their position, they inevitably argue for the stronger "what should be done" instead of the weaker "what may be done." Hence, the debate over the use of stem cells appears to be too normatively charged for either side to let the question linger in the moral "no man's land" of an arbitrariness with no political or legal warrant one way or the other.

In this chapter I argue for the prohibition of taking stem cells from a live embryo (which entails killing the embryo in the process). Without the argument that follows, I can only stipulate my normative conclusion here and now. As this chapter makes plain in due course, my mode of argumentation is philosophical, even though the texts on which I draw as illustrations in that argument are theological in that they are taken from the Jewish religious tradition, which is my primary locus in this world. Nevertheless, I do not invoke religious texts authoritatively here. My argument is not a responsum (a *teshuvah*, meaning an answer) or formal rabbinical response to a question asking for a ruling on the basis of classical Jewish sources: the Bible, the Talmud, and the codes. The argument I present here does not use the rhetoric that is used in the responsa literature (*she'elot u-teshuvot*).

To be sure, in my capacity as a rabbinical arbiter (*poseq*) I do respond to questions of Jewish law asked within the traditional Jewish community—specifically, the segment of the traditional Jewish community, however small, whose members from time to time authorize me to resolve their halakhic dilemmas (*she'elot*).[18] Finally, although I do not argue here in a strictly political way (which usually becomes legal argumentation before too long), one could draw at least some public policy implications from what I say here. Nevertheless, I do not make any specific public policy statements here because I am not a secular legislator, nor do I make any legal rulings because I am not a secular judge. I am only a theologically committed and morally interested citizen of the United States and Canada who makes his living as an academic philosopher and sometimes gets involved in debates of public philosophy. This self-identification, of course, gets to the interrelation of philosophy and politics. (The relations of theology to philosophy and politics are more complicated and thus are far more intelligible if the more evident interrelation of philosophy and politics is examined first.)

The relation of philosophy and politics is evident in the public arguments (however badly enunciated) of persons who exercise political authority and even for citizens who make their moral views known to these authorities. This relationship is evident in the realm of lawmaking whether the law is a prohibition or a mandate. Sometimes, moral prohibitions or moral injunctions that involve matters of great public concern and have considerable public support become new law. Consider, for example, how the moral prohibition of slavery became the law, so that slaveholding is now outlawed in almost every human society. Consider also how the moral injunction to treat women no differently from the way men are treated in public has led to new laws mandating gender equality in many civil societies. Thus, moral considerations lead to repeal of old positive law and engender new positive law. Philosophically formulated morality, which is morality argued for rationally rather than being derived from positive law, is logically prior to positive law because rational morality is the minimal criterion for old law to remain normative and the maximal standard for new law to become normative.

All official lawmakers (legislators) and judges who apply the law in normative judgments should be prepared to answer the questions every intelligent citizen should ask during great moral debates in society: Why should I obey the law you have made or now propose?

Why should I obey the law you are administering? Why should I obey your legal judgments? All of these public officials should be able to give some sort of philosophical argument for the moral position they are representing to the citizens of their society.

Minimally, old law should not contradict morality; if it does, it should be regarded retrospectively as human error and repealed. Maximally, new law should be made for moral reasons—which means replacing the particular legal decisions of previous legislators, administrators, and judges in a particular society with new ones and in the larger context of universal humanity discussed by philosophy. Through this process of recontextualization, these earlier decisions are shown to be morally inappropriate, or at least morally inappropriate in a changed social climate. As such, universal morality bespeaks a wider and deeper public domain than that bespoken by any system of positive law. Therefore, morality cannot be relegated to the realm of individual privacy, to become a matter of mere taste, which gives morality less public significance than it deserves. (Privacy could be defined as the realm of human existence that is too deprived of importance—a *privatio*—for society to bother to institute any public supervision of it in the form of law and legal penalty.) Hence, all significant moral questions inevitably wind up in the courts, the legislature, or the corridors of executive power—the places where justice as obligatory public order is decided or proposed. (The issue of whether the courts, the legislature, or the corridors of executive power are the primary locus of justice is hotly debated today, especially in Canada and the United States, and watching where conclusive treatment of issues such as the use of stem cells will be politically decided in these two countries will be interesting.) That is why, for Aristotle, justice (*dikaiosynē*) is the most important moral character trait to be cultivated by every rational person—that is, by all persons who understand that their rational and discursive capacity (*logos*) makes their participation in a worthy human realm (*polis*) possible.[19] Reason and justice intimately involve each other. Just as our capacity for reason makes intelligent and intelligible speech possible, our capacity for justice makes a respectable society and its law possible. Reason and justice are socially enabling. Reason is justifiable speech; justice is rational action.

In the following section, I take a more detailed look at the interrelation of philosophy, politics, and theology—especially the interrelation of philosophy and theology—so that we can better appreciate the theoretical issues involved in the question of stem cell research. Appreciation of these abstract theoretical issues will enable us to see how the method we use in deciding this practical issue is not confined to this issue alone; it can be used with regard to other such issues. We also can see that the practical treatment of this issue can illustrate how ethics is, in the words of the late-nineteenth/early-twentieth-century German-Jewish philosopher Hermann Cohen, "the theory of praxis."[20]

PHILOSOPHY, POLITICS, AND THEOLOGY AND THEIR INTERRELATIONS

Although philosophy, politics, and theology are interrelated, they bespeak different realms of human existence; hence, none of them should be reduced to the other. Furthermore, philosophy has a different relation to politics than it does to theology, and theology has a different relation to philosophy than it does to politics. Maintaining these different modes of relationality also is important to avoid confusion.

Philosophy is the proper context or forum for discussion of universal morality. Universal morality or natural law is what my philosophical mentor, Germain Grisez, once called "an intellect-size bite of reality."[21] Theology is the context for discussion of religious law. Politics is the context for discussion of secular positive law. Thus, assuming that every practical norm will be translated into positive law is a category error, a confusion of philosophy and politics or theology and politics. Consider the prohibition of the practice of homoeroticism, for example. Although there might be good religious grounds for prohibiting it (namely, specific biblical proscriptions) and good moral reasons for prohibiting it (it treats a male body as if it were female or a female body as if it were male; it takes its practitioners away from society's need for maximal family life), legally outlawing the behavior and empowering the government to penalize persons who engage in it by depriving them of their liberty (by imprisonment) or their property (by fining them) probably is imprudent politically. Enforcement of such a positive law surely would involve an invasion of the sexual privacy of consenting adults that most citizens in our society take for granted; hence, most citizens probably would resent the violation of privacy for any reason short of rescuing an unwilling victim of sexual assault. Moreover, such a positive law would be unlikely to have the support of enough citizens to condemn persons who violate it by designating them as outlaws. In fact, such a law might even create sympathy for homosexuals as members of a persecuted minority. (Consider how even moral condemnation of homoeroticism recently has been branded with the opprobrium "homophobia.")

Such political restraint is not called for, however, in the debate over stem cell research. Stem cell research is conducted in a laboratory, which is a public place—not in anyone's bedroom. Moreover, the most important person involved in stem cell research is the donor embryo, who is certainly not a consenting adult but the victim of an unjustified assault. As such, the question of stem cell research is not only appropriate for theology and philosophy; it also is a political question by virtue of its public character in secular societies.

With regard to theology, which is the proper context or forum for discussion of religious law, in my view it is essentially historical theology: the God-talk of a single historical community. Thus, when I use the term "theology" I mean the only theology that has a claim on me: Jewish theology (even though theology appears to function similarly in the revelation-based monotheistic faiths of Christianity and Islam). Theology is the forum in which a historical community represents God's revealed word to them, which they have received in faith. Hence, theology is not so much human talk about God as the reformulation of God's revelation to humans of their existential situation in the world. Theology is addressed to humans and calls for an active response from them, so it is essentially normative. It teaches what God requires of humans to live their lives in harmony with the way God has placed them in the world, which is to live purposeful lives with God and with each other.[22] Moreover, all talk about God becomes what God requires his people to say back to God. Thus, human God-talk is primarily liturgical (*lex orandi est lex credendi*); it speaks to God in the second person before we can speak about God in the third person because of what comes from God speaking in the first person: "I am the Lord your God" (Exodus 20:2).[23] Theological God-talk must not contradict what the worshiping community says to God, let alone what God says about Himself in relation to His people in revelation. By its formulation and reformulation of revelation, theology is constantly becoming revelation's transmitting tradition (*masoret*).

In its representation of the content of revelation, theology is formulated and reformulated through the persons the covenanted community designates to be its authoritative teachers (*hakhamim*). Within that ongoing transmission of the content of revelation, the community even regards itself as authorized to augment that revelation from time to time with innovations designed to protect the content of that revelation from gradual practical erosion or to further enhance what the community perceives to be the overall purposes of the law of God.[24] As law (*halakhah*), Jewish theology represents what God positively claims from the community covenanted with Him because He is their God. Alternatively, law is what the community's authorized representatives interpret those positive claims to be. Law also is what the community's authorized representatives add to those claims as if that very addition had been posited by God.[25]

Theology is addressed to the particular faith community, for that community. It is speech derived from God's word; it is not speech about God from humans reflecting on the world outside of revelation. Of course, because such theology is spoken in human language, it is intelligible to outsiders; indeed, humanity per se might be its ultimate addressee.[26] Nevertheless, theology cannot make valid normative claims upon anyone outside the community that speaks it, unless such an outsider is already becoming an insider through the process of religious conversion (*giyyur*).[27] Theology is not human speculation about God's relation to the cosmos independent of God's revelation to humans. Such speculation independent of revelation has been called "natural theology." Use of the term natural theology, however, is a category error that confuses theology with philosophy. Moreover, it asserts more than philosophy can cogently assert and less than theology can cogently assert, so it is neither, properly speaking. Natural theology cannot give philosophers an absolute with whom they can be philosophically concerned, and it cannot give members of a faith community such as Judaism the God they need to worship. Natural theology is a distraction from a philosopher's inability to speak of God at all philosophically, and it is a distraction from a theologian's ability to speak of the far richer God who presents Himself in revelation.[28]

Having clarified the essentially historical character of theology, one can understand why a secular society's fundamental warrant cannot come from any revelation and the tradition any revelational theology formulates. A secular society can remain secular only when it is multicultural—that is, when most of its citizens come from a variety of traditions, each of which is founded on a different revelation. To maintain its historically impartial secularity, however, any secular society must regard the truth claims of each of these revelation-founded traditions as having equal value. As such, it cannot regard any of them as its foundation because doing so would require the secular society to make a theological judgment—to utter a theological preference—by which it would thereby lose its secularity. Nevertheless, that indifference to specifically theological claims does not mean that a secular society can act as if the religious commitments of its various members are politically irrelevant or worthless or that they have been philosophically refuted. Doing so would create a social vacuum that inevitably would be filled by some new god for such a forgetful society.

When a secular society assiduously avoids public God-talk, even attempting to delegitimize such talk (as is increasingly happening in Canadian and U.S. politics and law), such a society is thereby unable to dispel any of its patriotic citizens from ascribing divinity or ultimacy to that society itself—especially to the state that governs that society—and most especially ascribing ultimate divinity to the sovereign who personifies that society. Indeed, that process of replacing the old God with a new god has been evident in modern Communism and in more virulent modern nationalisms such as Nazism.

Nevertheless, there can be no direct relation between theology and politics in the public discourse of such a society—only one of indirection, which is unlike the direct relation that does and should pertain between philosophy and politics there. (Contrast that relation with the intimate relation between theology and politics that obtained in ancient Israel—a point Spinoza recognized more clearly than any other philosopher.)[29] As such, any theological claims on a secular society must be mediated by philosophy. Thus, there might be a valid philosophical claim on a secular society such as that the law should prohibit the taking of any innocent human life, which also is an explicit religious command: "I am the Lord your God. . . . Thou shalt not kill" (Exodus 20:2, 13). In a secular society, however, only the philosophical claim can be publicly meaningful; the theological claim can be put forth only as one's personal religious motive for making the philosophical claim. (That personal motive is more than a private claim because it comes from one's personal commitment to a greater, not lesser, community than the secular state could possibly be and still remain secular.) Yet once the political distance of theology from politics is properly contrasted with the political proximity of philosophy, we can see theology having some benefit for philosophy (though never having to seek its warrant from philosophy), especially for philosophy that is directly related to the practical political concerns of social justice. First, however, let us see more precisely how philosophy and politics are to be related to each other and then see some more of what theology can actually do in and for a secular political order.

If one regards morality to be the minimal standard for positive law (*conditio sine qua non*), and if one regards moral obligation to be logically prior to legal obligation, then no positive law that contradicts morality is morally obligatory. No command should be obeyed when it is morally prohibited, even when it is legally prescribed.[30] One is a moral subject before (*a priori*) one is a subject of any legal system, even though one becomes aware (*a posteriori*) of one's legal subjectivity before one becomes aware of one's moral subjectivity. (For example, I obeyed my parents because of their legal power over me, discovering only later why their claims upon me were, in essence, right—that is, morally justified.)

Thus, we can see how philosophy is related to politics. How is theology related to moral philosophy, and why does philosophy need to acknowledge theology's presence in the world? We can see theology's relationship to ethics or practical wisdom (or moral philosophy) in four ways.

The first relation of theology to philosophy is negative in that theology functions as a brake on the metaphysical pretensions of philosophy. As such, in discussing the grounds of morality, philosophy can speak about human life as having a transcendent intention and that transcendence as the reason for its inviolability by all other creatures—a point well put by twentieth-century German philosopher Karl Jaspers.[31] (This intention is evidenced in the concern with God throughout humankind, whether they manifest it by seeking God or fleeing God.) Yet philosophy cannot and should not discuss what constitutes a real relationship with the transcendence human existence intends and thus what constitutes the core of unique human nature. In political debates, for example, when a philosophical position on an issue such as the use of stem cells is accused of being theological and therefore inadmissible in secular political discourse, a philosopher must show that his or her discourse is not theological, not just by denial but by showing what is authentic theological discourse by contrast.

One can set forth the limitations of any mode of discourse only by showing what is limiting it on the other side of its ultimate horizon.[32] By admitting the possibility of theological discourse about the God–human relationship—but without endorsing any particular theology as some sort of necessary conclusion from a philosophical reflection on the human condition—a philosopher can indicate that human nature intends transcendence without having to tell us what (or whom) human nature intends. Only when philosophers attempt to show the impossibility of theological discussion of the God–human relationship do theologians need to remind such philosophers that the only impossibility is logical absurdity. As long as a language is spoken coherently, one cannot claim that it has no grammar. Moreover, the fact that certain questions cannot be discussed cogently in one language form does not mean that these questions cannot be cogently discussed in another language form.

In its second relation to philosophy, theology functions positively for philosophy by providing a truly metaphysical context for the human quest for justice. Philosophy as ethics is surely needed to structure that striving so that it might truly become rational striving in the world. Yet philosophy cannot tell us anything about the true origin of that striving; it can only deny (*via negativa*) any substitutes for it. Philosophy can only indicate that our quest for justice seems to be a response to a transcendent claim; it cannot tell us who is making that claim upon us. At the other end of the cosmic spectrum, theology provides ethics and the moral striving it structures with an eschatological horizon. That is, theology reminds morally striving humans that their striving will lead to cynical despair if they think they can create any permanent good in the world, let alone cause justice to be finally accomplished in the world. Without this horizon, even the most dedicated moral idealist will inevitably conclude, "In place of justice [*ha-mishpat*] there is injustice [*ha-resha*]; in place of right is the wrongdoer [*ha-rasha*]" (Ecclesiastes 3:16). "He hoped for justice, but there is injustice [*mishpah*]; for righteousness [*tsedaqah*], but there is protest [*tse'aqah*]" (Isaiah 5:7). To counter this despair, theology explicates scriptural and traditional teachings of God as the ultimate Judge and Redeemer. These teachings are expressed in a human appeal to God such as Abraham's cry: "Will not the Judge of the whole earth do justice?" (Genesis 18:25). It also can be asserted in Job's assurance to himself and his helpless friends: "For I know that my Redeemer lives, even if He be the last to arise upon earth! Deep in my skin this has been marked, and with my own flesh I shall behold God" (Job 19:25–26).[33] Even a seemingly nontheological philosopher such as Kant saw the need for this kind of eschatology, although his own constitution of it suffers from his attempt to replace traditional eschatology with his own hybrid, postulated concoction.[34]

Theology, however, does not provide human moral striving with a God who will do the work of justice here and now in the world (a *Deus ex machina*) and who thus turns humans into merely passive spectators of a cosmic drama instead of active partners in that drama. Thus, this theology prevents overemphasis of God's role in cosmic justice by not substituting contemplation of God for covenantal praxis by humans.[35] Conversely, this theology prevents underemphasis of God's role by arguing that any substitute for God as the source and ultimate object of all moral law, such as human autonomy, is inadequate to our experience of moral law as commandment (*mitsvah*) from what is beyond identification with any of our own projects or ideals.[36] With morality, as with any other human endeavor, only God has the right to say, "I am the first; I am also [*af*] the last" (Isaiah 48:12).

In its third relation to philosophy, theology functions positively for philosophy by virtue of its historicity. The perennial questions with which philosophy, especially ethics, deals have a long history in traditions such as Judaism. For example, the philosophical question of rights, which some scholars have tried to show is a *novum* of modernity, has been shown by more careful scholars to have been discussed in premodern cultures—many of which are still alive and well today and seem to have an open future ahead of them.[37] Likewise, for this discussion concerning the ethical question of when human life deserving protection begins, the Jewish tradition provides some powerful precedents that invite adoption in our contemporary discussions and debates on this question of use of stem cells that kill the embryos from which they have been taken. Persons who are involved in secular debates about issues such as this can still see and learn from live discussion of such issues in a faith community such as Judaism (that is, when Jewish thinkers can represent these discussions with philosophical acuity).

To be sure, these theological precedents are not authoritative in a secular society. They cannot be used to govern, only to guide. They are suggestions, not decrees; a voice, not a veto. Yet the fact that the basic ethical question involved in the stem cell discussion and debate has been inherited rather than invented by secular modernity means that modern ethicists cannot claim to be reasoning *de novo*. Thus, they cannot pretend that the generic question has no older history of discussion, just as they cannot pretend that they themselves or those whom they are addressing have come from nowhere. They cannot claim to be engaging in universal discourse when they refuse to listen to voices from communities past and present that are beyond the narrow universe of their own making. Modern ethicists are entering a philosophical discussion they did not initiate and can never conclusively terminate. They need to listen—critically, to be sure—to thinkers who have more experience in dealing with these questions than recent, largely academic, discussion has had.

Nevertheless, theology is most helpful for philosophy when it philosophizes internally—that is, when it engages in philosophical argumentation within the internal moral discourse of the religious community whose theology it is. That is theology's fourth relation to philosophy.

The Jewish tradition recognizes a large degree of autonomy for the discipline of ethics itself. That autonomy, however, is not to be confused with what many modern ethicists mean by autonomy, which is the assumption that ethical subjects are their own law-givers—that they make their own law for themselves. (In the Kantian version of autonomy, an ethical subject also makes the law for himself or herself and all other similar rational beings.)[38] Instead, what this autonomy or independence of ethics means is that practical or moral reasoning can be conducted primarily through the proposition of and argument for rationally evident norms and principles. Autonomy is about the independence of moral law itself (*nomos autos*) from either theology or politics. It is not about the ethical subject, the acting person, as the origin of that law. To be sure, there also is interpretation and application of canonical, normative texts such as scripture and the Talmud within Jewish ethics. Nevertheless, even maximally, that interpretation and application almost always treat those texts as if they were conclusions from moral reason—conclusions that have been written down.[39] Minimally, Jewish ethicists need only avoid any direct contradiction of a canonical text—unless, of course, that canonical text is vague enough to be easily reinterpreted.

Theology certainly continues to ground Jewish ethics, but only in the sense that it enables moral conclusions to be considered part of divinely revealed law. Theology as reformulation of the revealed word of God does not provide a logical premise, however, from which one can deduce specific moral conclusions. At most, theology provides Jewish ethics with sufficient general authorization for Jewish ethicists to engage in their independent discipline without having to get specific authorization from theological texts for every moral judgment they make. Jewish ethicists, then, essentially have to direct their practical reasoning according to what they believe the universal ends of the law are.[40]

The autonomy of ethics as a discipline itself is evident in a very theological way in an important legal judgment of Maimonides (d. 1204)—for many people the greatest of all Jewish theologian-jurists. In setting a criterion for when one says the prescribed blessing before performing a commanded act (*birkat mitsvah*) and when one does not, Maimonides rules that one is to say the blessing before performing an act only when God is the direct object of the act (*bein adam le-maqom*).[41] For example, one says the blessing about God sanctifying the Sabbath (*qiddush*) as the expression of one's intention to keep the Sabbath because it is "a Sabbath for the Lord [*shabbat l'adonai*]" (Exodus 20:10).[42] Thus, the fifteenth-century commentator Joseph Karo astutely infers that one is not to say this blessing before performing any act whose object is a fellow human (*bein adam le-havero*).[43] That is, the invocation of God as the source of the commandment is not to be made when the act pertains to any human interaction or transaction, which is the subject matter of ethics. Yet isn't God, for Judaism, the source of all commanded acts?[44] Isn't God declared the blessed source "who sanctifies us by His commandments, commanding us to" do X or Y or Z?[45]

Surely a theonomous system such as Judaism cannot assert that the human subject of the commanded act is also its source, that he or she is commanding himself or herself autonomously. So what difference does it make whether the object of the commanded act is human or divine if God is the source of the act anyway? Maimonidean commentators do not seem to address this theological question. Nevertheless, a phenomenological explanation might help us see what the essence of Jewish ethics is—indeed, what the essence of any ethics could be—and the philosophical significance of its operative autonomy. This phenomenology might better explain, among other things, how Maimonides could make such good use of so much Aristotelian ethical theory and so much Platonic political theory in his theorizing and even his practical application of Jewish morality.

In ethically significant action, wherein the direct object of the act is a human being, to do the act directly for the sake of God would be to ignore the immediate need of the human object before us: the one who is claiming us here and now. Consider a would-be murder victim who asks not to be killed. Think of someone in danger who asks a bystander to save him or her from harm. Think of a starving person who asks for bread.[46] That claiming person is the direct object of the commandment (which can be given in the form of a request when the subject of the command is willing to hear it). If one takes ethics as a discipline of rationally validating or justifying appropriate interhuman claims (and, conversely, rationally invalidating inappropriate ones), the justifiable or ethically validated claim of a human claimant on his or her fellow human being also is the direct source of the commanded act. Such an ethically validated claim should be obvious to the rational persons who are the subjects of the commandments. That is why such claims are immediate. At this point, God is more remote: He is the ultimate source of the ethically commanded act. God also is the ultimate end of any ethically commanded act inasmuch as the human object of the act has a claim upon us ultimately because he or she is the image of God (*tse-lem elohim*).

Accordingly, God's commandment that "you shall not murder" (Exodus 20:13) stands behind—in the background, as it were—the would-be victim's claim (even if the claim is made only through his or her body language), "Please, do not kill me!" God's commandment that "you shall not stand idly by the blood of your neighbor" (Leviticus 19:16) stands behind the would-be victim's claim, "Please save me!"[47] The needs of that other person, expressed through his or her justifiable claims on others to satisfy those needs (as best they can), are the subject matter of ethics.[48] Those needs should be the sole determinant of what is to be done for that person. Invoking God as the ultimate source of the commandment—which is the duty in response to the rightful claim of the human claimant—would be a distraction from the undivided attention that fulfillment of this commanded duty requires.[49]

The phenomenological independence of ethics from theology might indicate most clearly how ethics is the way "the Torah speaks according to human language."[50] That is especially so when rational human discussion of normative issues is taken as the superlative exercise of human language. In other words, Jewish normative discourse is most human when it discusses matters that are human per se. That is why Jewish discussion of universally human issues such as the use of embryonic stem cells is best conducted according to the criteria of ethics or moral reason. Along these lines, Israel Lipschuetz, a great Polish-Jewish rabbinic exegete of the nineteenth century, explained how normative Jewish ethics is distinct from Jewish ritual law: "The Torah permits human reason [*la-sekhel ha'enoshi*] to soar by its own strength, to analyze, enquire, and determine by its own sights . . . to weigh and judge according to its own reason . . . human reason has the ability to be quite precise in its intention of the final truth [*matarat ha'emet*] in any matter, over and above the fact that it has been obligated [by the Torah] to do so."⁵¹ That analysis appears to indicate that Jewish ethics is best conducted within (or, at least, alongside) the ethical and philosophical debates taking place in society at large. In the case of stem cell research, that discussion necessarily becomes political because it is a public policy issue; in fact, proponents are actively looking for public funding for such research, using all the tactics of political lobbying.

This excursus about the interrelations of theology, philosophy, and politics is important for this discussion. The discussion of philosophy is important to show how an issue such as stem cell research is most properly, and most productively, a question of moral reason. The discussion of theology is important to show Jews (and adherents of other religions of revelation, by analogy) that the philosophical treatment of a question such as stem cell research is not Jewishly disingenuous. In fact, similar philosophical discussions have already taken place within the Jewish tradition, which Jewish theology is constantly formulating and reformulating. The discussion of politics is important to remind both philosophers and theologians that no matter how cogent their philosophical or theological arguments about an issue such as stem cell research might be, their conclusions can and should only influence positive lawmaking, public policy, and adjudication; they should not expect these political institutions to implement them in toto. Thus, looking for a literal political translation of what has been ethically justified is not always politically possible or prudent.

THE STATUS OF THE EMBRYO
IN CURRENT JEWISH DISCUSSION

The main question—in fact, the only original moral question—concerning embryonic stem cell research is whether the week-old embryo has human status. Is the embryo a human person in any way? Does it have even the most minimal of human rights—the right not to be killed? Many scientists tell us that the cells from a week-old embryo are of optimal pluripotent quality—that is, they have the best chance of developing new tissue in another organism into which they have been injected. If the embryo does have human status, isn't destroying its chance to develop toward birth and beyond a violation of the basic rational norm—that another person is not to be harmed (*alterum non laedere*)?[52] Isn't that so even when one can derive substances from this embryo that would save or enhance another human life? Even in a case such as this, wouldn't there be a violation of the basic moral norm that "one life is not to be set aside for another" (*ein dohin nefesh mipnei nafesh*)?[53] Surely that is because of the principle that every human life is considered to be "a complete world itself" (*olam mal'e*), as the rabbis put it.[54] Kant wrote that every human life is an "end-in-itself" (*Zweck an sich selbst*) and is never to be used as a mere means for the benefit of another life—certainly not as a means to save another life that requires the sacrifice of one's own life.[55]

If one may not use embryonic stem cells for research, even if that research has a strong possibility of being a means to save other (even many) human lives, we could say that one ought not use them. On the other hand, if the week-old embryo does not have human status, one may use it for the sake of saving or even enhancing another human life. In fact, if its life-saving or life-enhancing status can be demonstrated, or even shown to be likely, one could invoke a moral obligation—an *ought*—in such a case. That is, one could say that one ought to use stem cells for life-saving or life-enhancing research. One might even say that every fertile male and female couple ought to provide the necessary biological materials for procreating an embryo to be used for stem cell research, in much the same way we say that everyone who is physically able has a moral obligation to donate his or her blood to a blood bank for the sake of saving other lives.

I take issue with many of my fellow Jewish ethicists—even some of those who affirm the Torah as the normative word of God and the traditional Jewish law (*halakhah*) as its authorized interpretation and application, as I do.[56] A philosophical or natural law reading of the traditional sources truly differs from a nonphilosophical or non–natural law position—what could be called legal positivism. This approach entails being guided by rational moral criteria and using current scientific knowledge in reading the few traditional sources that seem to pertain to this question. Although the specific question regarding the use of stem cells is novel, it is part of the more general issue of abortion, which shows no sign of being "finally settled"—as the famous headline of the *New York Times* on January 23, 1973, asserted the day after the U.S. Supreme Court's ruling in *Roe v. Wade* that permitted elective abortion when decided "by a woman and her doctor." (With the proliferation of abortion clinics, there has been little chance that a willing woman would not find a willing doctor to concur with her lethal decision, even if her decision could have been considerably influenced by a husband, a male partner, a parent, a peer group, or even general social approval and encouragement.)

Does the use of embryonic stem cells and the resulting death of the embryo as an independent human organism constitute an abortion or not? On this question there is an important difference between traditionalist and nontraditionalist Jewish ethicists (whom I call liberal rather than secular inasmuch as some of them consider themselves religious).

Almost all liberal Jewish ethicists have essentially accepted the secular liberal opinion that abortion is a woman's right, to be exercised for any reason whatsoever. In this view, the embryo (usually a fetus, given that most abortions take place in the third month of pregnancy) has no rights at all inasmuch as the only right it could possibly have at this early stage of its human development is its negative right not to be killed and its positive right to be nurtured by those who have conceived it. In this view, the embryo, and even the fetus, may be destroyed at will. Most of these Jewish ethicists, however, do draw the line at birth. Nevertheless, considering their proprietary view of the life of one's offspring, it is difficult to see how liberal ethicists of any kind can draw the line at birth with any cogency. In other words, it is hard to see how drawing any line later than the moment of conception itself is not purely arbitrary. Surely the difference between the vital independence of an embryo, a fetus, or an infant is a matter of degree rather than kind, as anyone who knows a nursing mother can easily recognize.

To their credit, most religious Jewish ethicists have resisted this liberal temptation to deny fetal or embryonic rights.[57] No one who is committed to the normative Jewish tradition could possibly say that there is a right to abortion.[58] The only warrant for an abortion is when the fetus—even the embryo—poses a direct threat to the life of the woman in whose body it is now living. Under these circumstances, the abortion is considered to be an act of self-defense by the mother. Surely it is irrational to expect any person to host somebody else within her own body who, if left there, is very likely to kill her. This situation is as if the fetus is in mortal pursuit (*kerodef*) of its own mother.[59] Saving one's own life takes precedence over saving the life of someone else when only one life can be saved.[60] With regard to third parties, they have the duty to save the human life most proximate to them, which by definition will always be the life of the mother because the life of the fetus or embryo, in utero, is always more remote from everybody—even the woman who is carrying it—compared to the mother's own life.[61] (I discuss the pertinent classical Jewish texts on these points shortly.)

At this point, the only debate among the traditionalists is how widely or narrowly to draw the circle around what constitutes an imminent threat to the present human life of the mother. Moreover, we can assume that the imminent threat to maternal life is not pregnancy per se, which does involve some *possible* risks to any pregnant woman but poses more *probable* risks to very few pregnant women today.[62] Nevertheless, the burden of proof is always on the woman who requests an abortion for herself or on the third party requesting an abortion for her. Without such proof of the need for what is, in effect, a dispensation from the prohibition of bloodshed (*shefikhut damim*), the prohibition stands.[63] That is, the presumption (*hazaqah*) of the right to life always inheres in the fetus or even the embryo. The burden of proof is on the accuser—

that is, the person who claims something contrary to the usual state of affairs.[64] No one is required to prove anything to protect prenatal life. It is a *prima facie* right—albeit a right that its bearer cannot exercise for himself or herself; it must be exercised on his or her behalf by others, who are obligated by the norm "thou shalt not stand idly by the blood of your neighbor" (Leviticus 19:16), which is the rationally evident duty to rescue somebody else from death or even from any lesser harm. The question is: Who is my neighbor? When does human life obtain its most basic personal right, its most basic claim on all others—not to be killed and to be nurtured so it can continue to grow until God takes that human life back?

If the prohibition of abortion (and the warrant for abortion of a fetus that threatens the life of his or her mother) is to be something Jewish thinkers can enter into the current philosophical debate over embryonic stem cell research, the prohibition (and the warrant) must be represented as the discovery of Judaism, not the invention of Judaism. Even if the subjects of the prohibition (and the warrant) are taken to be all humankind, there is no reason for any non-Jew to accept either the prohibition or the warrant simply because the Jewish tradition says so. In other words, only when the Jewish tradition can represent such prohibitions and warrants rationally rather than prescribing them do the prohibition and the warrant have enough universal validity to be given to all rational persons who are ethical subjects on behalf of all persons (even those who are prerational, such as fetuses, or postrational, such as persons who are senile or irreversibly comatose) who are ethical objects.

Nevertheless, when Jews (or members of any religion with a revealed law) represent any such prohibition or warrant as the invention of human reason rather than its discovery, are such Jews (or Christians or Muslims) not designating a source of their morality that stands apart from and in contrast to the law of God they proclaim (at least to themselves and to God) to be the source of their morality? Of course, that is what most liberal Jewish thinkers do when they deny the Jewish dogma of the divine revelation of the Torah (*torah min ha-shamayim*) by presuming that the Torah is a human invention, albeit an "inspired" one.

To overcome this dilemma, we must see how natural law in Judaism is the Jewish discovery of the law of God as it applies to all humankind—law that also is discoverable by any rational human being. Human reason or wisdom is primarily heuristic; only divine wisdom is primarily creative or autonomous, in the strong sense of that term. Furthermore, as the discovery of divine law, human reason can discover only the aspect of divine law that is necessary for a decent human life in a decent human society; it cannot discover the fuller aspect of divine law that is by itself sufficient for a communal life whose members are truly aware of their place in the cosmos by virtue of their direct covenantal relationship with God. That awareness or apprehension can come only from historical revelation—when God, as it were, discovers humankind in the covenanted community, in the people God has elected to be His portion in the world. Thus, the discovery of natural law by Jews is not displacement of divine wisdom with human invention; nor does the discovery of natural law displace revealed divine law, which must be given to humans but which they can never obtain by their own efforts, however sublime.

NATURAL LAW IN JUDAISM

To better understand how a philosophically persuasive position on embryonic stem cell research can be formulated by Jewish theologians for the world, we should first see how such a position can be formulated by Jewish theologians for Jews. We need to see how natural law thinking operates within Judaism and then see how it operates for the world. We need to see theologically why this way of doing practical reason is endemic within the Jewish tradition and is not simply apologetics—that is, it does not operate with some sort of dual-truth ethical epistemology: one for Jews and another for non-Jews.[65]

Jewish tradition recognizes that the Torah did not come into a normative vacuum: The people Israel were already living under an earlier law before the revelation at Mount Sinai. That law is what the rabbis called the seven Noahide commandments (*sheva mitsvot bnei Noah*).[66] For purposes of ethical enquiry, pertaining to the realm of interhuman relationships, the pertinent norms to consider are the prohibitions of shedding the blood of innocents (*shefikhut damim*); robbery (*gezel*); and sexual immorality (*gilui arayot*), which includes prohibitions of incest, adultery, homosexuality, and bestiality. There also is one positive norm: the injunction to any lawful society to establish a system of justice (*dinim*)—what we now call due process of law. This norm denotes a system of justice that provides systematic administration and adjudication of the other six Noahide commandments. Hence, in cases involving violations of the three foregoing ethical prohibitions, we could say that the system of justice is to adjudicate violations of human bodies (the most severe being bloodshed), human property, and the human family.

Some theologians have regarded Noahide law as an earlier form of positive law—that is, law specifically posited or directly proclaimed by God's command.[67] As such, this earlier law differs from the later Mosaic law in degree rather than kind. Both are directly revealed divine decrees, but Noahide law obligates all humankind at all times, whereas Mosaic law (Torah, both written and oral; the Law, both scriptural and traditional) obligates only Jews after the Sinai revelation. Indeed, after the Sinai revelation, Noahide law obliges non-Jews only, although the Mosaic law that comes after Noahide law does not repeal any of it but merely repeats it and supplements it. The question, however, is whether Mosaic law is more than a supplement to Noahide law and whether Noahide law is more than a historical introduction to Mosaic law. Does either law do anything for the other or not?

Other theologians have regarded the difference between Noahide law and Mosaic law as a difference in kind. Whereas Mosaic law is the direct decree of God, given to a single human community at a certain point in history, Noahide law is not the direct decree of God but a rational human inference that God stands behind norms that seem to oblige all humans at all times. These commandments, especially, have been most often called rational commandments (*mitsvot sikhliyot*).[68] They are the equivalent of what has been called natural law (*ius naturale*), which is law discovered by humans when they rationally discern the authentic needs and justifiable claims of their human nature. To use Kantian language, one could say of this view that whereas Mosaic law is known from historical experience *a posteriori*, Noahide law is known retrospectively *a priori*. That is, after noting that some basic norms seem to be both international and pre-Mosaic, we can discern why. We can infer that this generality is not accidental; it has a universal reason. These generally extant norms must be affirmed and administered by any human society that makes claims upon its members as rational and free human persons, whose basic rights and duties come from a source that transcends the power of any human society in the world, no matter how powerful or wise. A society affirms natural law when it recognizes in its positive law and public policies that the human persons who live in that society or come into contact with it in any way have an essentially transcendent orientation that makes them inviolable.

Asserting that natural law is discovered rather than invented by human reason means that natural law is not a displacement of divine law; it is the singularly rational discovery of divine law in its most universal manifestation. Therefore, acceptance of natural law is not at odds with acceptance of divine law; it is the beginning of human acceptance of divine law. "Happy is the human person [*adam*] who has found wisdom" (Proverbs 3:13). Indeed, initial human acceptance of natural law through human reason makes acceptance of the more ample aspect of divine law, which can only be revealed, superrational rather than irrational. A lawless, irrational mob would have been in no position to cogently accept the Torah. To go beyond human reason rather than beneath it requires one to go through human reason.

The difference between the two forms of divine law is that natural law is discovered by human reason within its experience of human life as naturally communal—specifically, through the rightful claims humans make on each other, collectively and individually. Assuming that natural law comes from divine creative wisdom is to give an irreducible metaphysical reason for the justifiable human claims that deserve to be codified into positive law. Revealed law, on the other hand, is God's way of directly claiming human beings for a positive relationship with Himself, even if that relationship at present can be with only one people in the world.

The Torah is the perpetual gift (*mattan torah*) resulting from "God in search of man," in the words of my late revered teacher, Abraham Joshua Heschel.[69] It is how humans are able to live a covenanted life with God in the world. Moreover, it enables humans to patiently anticipate the final redemption (*ge'ulah*) of Israel, humankind, and the cosmos itself, because through revealed divine law humans have already experienced a small part of that final redemption already.[70]

Natural law prepares us to accept revealed law precisely because it is preparation for but not identical with a fully significant human life in the world. As such, by its existential insufficiency, natural law induces in us the desire to receive directly from God what our proper and concrete location in the universe is truly meant to be and how we are to fully dwell there until the end of days (*ahareet ha-yamim*). What revealed law lacks in universality it gains in intensity. Thus, one might take redemption (*ge'ulah*) to be the historical end-time when the abstract universality of natural law and the concreteness of historically revealed law will merge into one everlasting eschatological realm.[71]

Notwithstanding the difference in kind between these two forms of divine law, they are closely related. This greater closeness is evident in the Talmud's enunciation of this principle: "There is nothing permitted [*shar'ei*] to the Jews that has been prohibited [*asur*] to the non-Jews."[72] In the positivist view, there is no reason to assert this principle. If Mosaic law is only a supplement or even a further development of Noahide law, why can't Mosaic law repeal—that is, radically change—the earlier (in effect, more "primitive") law?[73] Yet when one takes Noahide law as natural law to be *a priori* and thus universal, it is much more than a mere supplement to—even more than the potential of—*a posteriori* Mosaic law. Because Noahide law is *a priori*, acceptance of Mosaic law is possible for rational human beings. Yet Mosaic law is not derived from Noahide law, nor does it merely specify it further. Instead, Mosaic law need only not contradict Noahide law. Moreover, like a Kantian *a priori* condition or precondition for experience, Noahide law and its principles ever accompany Mosaic law, as our innately temporal consciousness always accompanies every timely experience it makes possible for us.[74] In fact, natural or Noahide law is always available to counteract the temptation of some Jewish theologians to make Jewish law fanatical, chauvinistic, or inhumane.

When Mosaic law adds to Noahide law, it does so specifically and generally. With regard to the basic moral norms of Noahide law, Mosaic law in effect repeats them rather than changing or repealing them. Mosaic law has much more content. Actual differences between the two forms of divine law governing interhuman relationships lie only in the area of criminal penalties for violations of norms that are common to Noahide and Mosaic law.[75] The general supplementation of Noahide law by Mosaic or Jewish law, where Jewish law presents something totally new (*hiddush*), is in the area of the God–human relationship. It includes proscriptions or prohibitions for Jews regarding things such as working on the Sabbath or eating pork and prescriptions regarding things such as sanctifying the Sabbath by various rituals and eating unleavened bread (*matsah*) on Passover.[76] Despite this difference, however, even in the area of the God–human relationship Noahide law often functions as a minimal condition—what one contemporary Jewish theologian has called "a standard below which the demands of revelation could not possibly fall."[77] Thus, if one regards the duty to rescue an endangered human life as part of the Noahide law prohibiting bloodshed (which would be violated by omission if one did not rescue someone when one could do so short of sacrificing one's own life by so doing), then that duty is all the more the Jewish law.[78]

THREE RABBINIC TEXTS PERTAINING TO ABORTION

I now examine the Noahide prohibition of abortion within its proper normative context. Only then can we properly deal with the question of the use of embryonic stem cells, which seems to be a subset of this prohibition. I look at three rabbinic texts (and their biblical roots) that have sometimes been misinterpreted; that misinterpretation has led to some erroneous conclusions regarding the use of pluripotent stem cells. The misinterpretations and misconceptions they involve also can be cleared up through a legitimate reading of all such texts that deal with interhuman relations from a natural law perspective. That perspective performs a heuristic function in reading the classical texts on this overall issue. We need to read these texts as assertions resulting from moral reasoning—assertions that require us to read them rationally, the same way they were written. We need to read them philosophically.

The first text is the most explicit prohibition of abortion in the rabbinic sources. It is an exegesis (*midrash*) of the scriptural verse "whosoever sheds human blood [*dam ha'adam*] by humans [*ba'adam*] shall his blood be shed because in the image of God He made humankind [*ha'adam*]" (Genesis 9:6).[79] I explore what this verse means in its own scriptural context to allow us to better appreciate what the rabbis did with it in their exegesis.

Given that this text mentions the punishment for the crime of murder, we can infer that murder has already been prohibited. The reason for the severe punishment is not just that the punishment should fit the crime, as in "a life for a life" (Exodus 21:23; Leviticus 24:18), but that killing another human being also is taken to be an indirect assault on God.[80] Thus, the preceding verse states, "I shall reckon [*edrosh*] your life-blood from the hand of every beast I shall reckon it, and from the hand of humans [*ha'adam*]: from a man's brother I shall reckon the human life [*nefesh ha'adam*]" (Genesis 9:5). The reader of this verse probably is expected to remember how God avenged the death of Abel, who was murdered by his brother Cain—both of whom were the first humans created in the image of God through normal conception and birth. God indicts Cain for the murder of his only human peer (Adam and Eve having been created by God but not having been born in the natural way)—a punishment about which Cain complains, "my punishment [*avoni*] is too great to bear!" (Genesis 4:13). How was Cain expected to know that what he did to his brother is prohibited—that it was something for which he is then to be punished? Can a punishment be just when the criminal did not know in advance that what he was about to do is wrong (*nulla poena sine lege*)?[81] Where has scripture previously told us of a prohibition of murder?

The answer seems to be that Cain and Abel were both expected to be aware of the fact that they had been created in the image of God (*tselem elohim*). As such, an assault on the image is tantamount to an assault on the One whose image has been assaulted. The difference is that an assault on the image is effective; an assault on the One standing behind that image is ineffective.[82] Hence, the One whose image has been assaulted can always punish the assailant; the victim cannot take revenge on the assailant but can only have this revenge effected for him or her.

How did Cain and Abel know they are the image of God? Moreover, even if they did know that, how could such a fact lead to a norm? Indeed, as David Hume most famously argued, an *ought* cannot be derived logically from an *is*.[83] One possible answer to this question comes from the verse that describes the first contact God made with the first humans: Adam and Eve, the parents of Cain and Abel. "And the Lord God commanded the humans [*al ha'adam*]" (Genesis 2:16). Although "the humans" seem to be the subjects of the verb "command," the rabbis interpret the preposition *al* ("on") to also literally designate the objects of the verb: "The Lord God commanded *concerning* humans"—that is, what may or may not be done to them.[84] By this exegesis, the rabbis assume that the verse is the original version of "thou shalt not murder."[85] In other words, humans become aware that they—I and you—are the image of God (a fact of which the readers of scripture have already been informed by Genesis 1:26–27) when they become aware of themselves as the unique subjects of divine commands, in that they are the only creatures who are freely aware enough to either obey or disobey these commands. As such, humans are both the unique subjects and the unique objects of divine command. Divine command is itself God's concern inasmuch as the first command is a beneficent warning to humans about how to avoid death: "On the day you eat from it [the tree of the knowledge of good and evil] you shall surely die" (Genesis 2:17).[86]

Command (*mitsvah*) or law (*ius*) has human subjects only. Accordingly, this notion must be taken metaphorically in connection with anything that does not show itself to have freedom of choice.[87] Of all creatures, only humans manifest freedom of choice (*liberum arbitrium*)—that is, the option to draw near to or avoid other beings or to treat those other beings well or badly.[88]

The image of God does not denote some sort of divine quality God partially transfers to humans; it indicates that humans are capable of a mutual relationship with the source of their existence in the world. That relationship is essentially normative—what scripture subsequently calls a covenant (*berit*).[89] How do we first hear these divine commands? How does God make His claims upon His unique creatures, created in His image? After all, the Torah as the Law has not yet been revealed. Perhaps, however, the original command of God—which can be taken to be "thou shalt not murder"— might be mediated by the would-be victim of the murderer. In other words, the command "thou shalt not murder" not only concerns humans (who are the only objects of murder, at least for nonvegetarians); it also is revealed through humans by virtue of being first uttered by humans. The very presence of one human being to another, even when hidden from immediate view, makes a normative claim upon any other human being who has the power to either harm or help. When asked who is making this claim upon us, the would-be victim can say (or have said on his or her behalf by a concerned human third party), "I am the image of God. An assault on me is an attempted assault on God, which is wrong in and of itself. What right does a creature have to assault his or her Creator? Furthermore, it is an attempted assault on God that God will not let go unpunished."

Here we are not deriving an *ought* from an *is*, at least not in the usual sense. Instead, the very "*is*-ness" or being or presence-in-the-world of that other person is itself an *ought* (which twentieth-century French-Jewish philosopher Emmanuel Levinas described with great phenomenological insight).[90] Our first experience of any other human person is that that person's very presence demands that we notice him or her—minimally by not harming the person, maximally by helping the person. Only the presence of nonpersons makes no immediate claim upon us—that is, their "*is*-ness" or being does not itself present an *ought* or a claim.[91] Therefore, a respect for the nonhuman world is best justified when we become aware of how God has given us that world to care for it and for ourselves in it and over it: "to work it and guard it" (Genesis 2:15); how God created the world "not to be a wasteland but to be a dwelling-place [*la-shevet*]" (Isaiah 45:18); and how "the earth has been given to humankind" (Psalms 115:16).[92]

The prohibition of killing the innocent in Genesis 9:6 is presupposed rather than directly proscribed, and even the punishment set down for such killing is not a direct prescription. "By humans shall his blood be shed [*yishafekh*]" is written in the less direct third-person form (what is to be done) rather than in the more direct second-person form (what you should do). Thus, the punishment is assumed rather than immediately commanded. Indeed, this indirect rather than direct commandedness characterizes the Noahide laws as the rabbis understood them. Therefore, the implied Noahide prohibition of bloodshed had to be repeated as "thou shalt not murder" by the Mosaic Torah (Exodus 20:13; Deuteronomy 5:17) to be a commandment (*mitsvah*) in the full covenantal sense for Jews.[93] That does not mean that the prohibition of murder was not binding and known to be binding before the Mosaic revelation; it simply means that before that direct revelation of God's fuller law, the prohibition of killing innocent human life was the commandment of the "hidden God" (Isaiah 45:15) rather than the commandment of the God "who arrived at Sinai . . . who appeared at Mount Paran" (Deuteronomy 33:2)—the God from whom "Moses commanded us the Torah" (Deuteronomy 33:4).[94] In fact, Genesis 9:6 is a re-presentation of a norm that has no single historical origin but is coterminous with human being in the world, at all times and everywhere. It is *a priori* in the sense that there is no time when a morally astute person could assume that this norm does not obtain—although, of course, it often is violated in practice and even mandated by positive laws such as those enacted in rogue polities such as Nazi Germany or Maoist China.

Now we can better appreciate the rabbinic exegesis of this verse, which brings in the issue of abortion: "Rav Jacob bar Aha found written in a book of Rav's dicta [*sefer aggadata*] that a Noahide is capitally liable . . . Rabbi Ishmael said even [for killing] fetuses [*af ha'ubarin*]. What is Rabbi Ishmael's rationale? It is written: 'Whosoever sheds human blood, by humans shall his blood be shed' (Genesis). Who is 'a human within a human [*adam ba'adam*]'? That is the fetus [*ubar*] in his mother's womb."[95] In other words, *ba'adam* ("by humans") refers not to the human judges who are to execute murderers but to a human life that is still contained within another human life—that is, the body of his or her mother.[96]

Again, the verse is not being interpreted to make a new prescription; it is interpreted to state an accepted fact that human life begins at conception, and killing it at any stage of its intrauterine development is tantamount to murder. The norm itself is alluded to by the scriptural verse (*asmakhta*) rather than literally derived from it.[97] As a description of a normatively significant fact, it is similar to the definition of human life described by the words of scripture, "The Lord God . . . breathed into his nostrils the breath of life [*nishmat hayyim*]" (Genesis 2:7)—which is taken to mean that human life is still human as long as its human subject is still breathing.[98] Undoubtedly, this statement also was already a universally accepted truth by the time the words of scripture describing it were actually written down.

Finally, this allusive function of scripture in relation to norms that are already known and accepted arises in a famous text of Maimonides. In discussing a Noahide who has kept the Noahide commandments as divine law rather than as merely wise counsels that just as easily could have been devised by humans, Maimonides writes, "He has accepted them and practiced them because of what God commanded [*mipnei she-tsivah ha-qadosh-barukh-hu*] concerning them in the Torah, which were made known to us through Moses our master, namely, that the Noahides had originally [*mi-qodem*] been commanded concerning them."[99] This text has been the topic of much intense debate since it was written in the twelfth century.[100] Contrary to much opinion (both pro- and anti-Maimonidean), however, Maimonides is not saying that Noahides—namely, humankind per se—have to derive their moral norms from the text of the Mosaic Torah to observe Noahide law as divine law. Not all divine law—that is, divinely given law (*torah*)—has to be derived from the text of historical revelation.[101] Maimonides is saying that the Torah is essentially describing or representing the divine law that already obtains for all humankind. Moses adds to it the norms God has specifically designated for Israel as a community whose national identity and constitution emerge simultaneously at the event of Sinai, when the fuller Torah is revealed.[102]

In fact, one can derive from various narratives in Genesis all of the Noahide commandments. For example, when Joseph resists the illicit advances of Potiphar's wife, he reminds her that the assignation she is inviting would be for both of them "a sin against God" (Genesis 39:9); that is, he assumes that she knows as well as he does that adultery is a sin against God and not just betrayal of her husband.[103] Thus, the rabbis interpreted the description of the founding of family life in the case of the first couple, Adam and Eve: "A man shall cleave to his wife [*b'ishtto*]" (Genesis 2:24)—from which one can infer, as Rabbi Akivah put it, "your wife but not someone else's wife [*eshet havero*]."[104]

Divine law is a genus with at least two species. The first species of divine law is the law that is discovered by human reason, which is coterminous with the presence of humankind in the world. The second species of divine law is the law Moses brought down from Mount Sinai for the sake of the people who had made him their agent to do just that for them. That is why Jews can speak of the first kind of divine law as natural law to the non-Jewish world and not thereby require non-Jews to accept Jewish moral authority. Jews are neither the source of natural law nor even its uniquely qualified interpreters. In other words, the Jewish representation of Noahide law to the world does not privilege Jews either theologically or politically. It simply gives Jews a rich history of philosophical reflection to draw upon and share with others.

Nevertheless, assuming Genesis 9:6 to be a literal prescription rather than a more general representation of what is usually the case could easily lead to the following inference: Because the text refers to human life in utero, perhaps human life created extra utero does not fall under the ban on abortion expressed in the words "within a human" (*ba'adam*). Embryonic stem cells are taken from an embryo that has been conceived through in vitro fertilization. That is, an ovum is taken from a woman's body, and some sperm are taken from a man's body; the two are fertilized in a laboratory in a petri dish. Whereas some embryos that are procreated through in vitro fertilization are meant to live and develop to term after being inserted into a woman's womb (usually the womb of the same woman from whom the eggs were taken), however, procreating embryos for the sole purpose of lethally deriving stem cells from them intends nothing but their death. Even people who are opposed to in vitro fertilization on moral grounds because it allows some of the fertilized embryos to die (because not all of them are reinserted in utero) would have to admit that the sin of commission involved in the derivation of stem cells is greater than this sin of omission, which only lets some of the fertilized embryos die because they couldn't all be reinserted in utero and be expected to live.[105] Nevertheless, one can avoid this entire issue by assuming that there are no moral norms governing what is done with what are now taken to be laboratory materials.

Following this literal exegesis, some theologians have suggested that only an embryo literally in utero could be the object of an illicit abortion.[106] Indeed, the same logic has been used to permit artificial insemination, even from an anonymous donor and even for a woman who is already married to another man. In this case too, conception of the embryo does not take place by means of a literal act of sexual congress; instead, sperm from the male donor is artificially inserted into the womb of the woman to be impregnated. The male and female bodies never come in contact with each other, and each can be totally anonymous to the other.[107]

Nevertheless, taking Genesis 9:6 to be a literal prescription—which it is not—and specifically qualifying it when it is meant to be interpreted generally, such clever overspecification (*pilpul*) might be appropriate in dealing with some very particular cases via casuistry. It is not appropriate, however, in suggesting major decisions regarding public policy. These decisions are made more appropriately when broad moral norms and ethical principles are the basis of the arguments for them and the exegesis of scriptural and traditional texts is designed to illustrate them.[108] What we see from the traditional Jewish treatment of Genesis 9:6 is that the discussion is conceptual rather than purely exegetical. Following this tendency, "inside a human" (*ba'adam*) should be taken to refer to the usual though not absolutely necessary place where an embryo or fetus is to be found.[109] As such, it also can include an embryo whose vital matrix is from the womb and whose conception is meant to be returned to the womb—that is, if the embryo has been conceived for life and not for death. Furthermore, the rabbis recognize at least two other situations where conception takes place outside of normal male-female sexual intercourse, yet one could not infer from these unusual occurrences that the product of this extra-uterine conception forfeits its most basic human right: the right to life.[110]

The notion that even the embryo in utero has human status and therefore is subject to all the protections of human life required by rational morality seems to be called into question by the second rabbinic text pertaining to the topic at hand: "The woman who is in hard-labor [*meqashah lailed*]: the fetus [*ha-vlad*] in her womb is to be dismembered and removed limb by limb because [*mipnei*] her life takes precedence over its life [*hayyav*]. But if most of it [the fetus] has already exited [the birth canal], then nothing is to be done to it [*ein nog'in bo*], for one life [*nefesh*] is not to be set aside [*ein dohim*] for another life."[111]

Some interpreters have used the comment of the great medieval exegete, the eleventh-century French rabbi known as Rashi (Rabbi Solomon Yitshaqi)—who is considered to be the greatest of the commentators on the Talmud—to draw an erroneous conclusion from this text. Rashi states that the reason for permitting—even mandating—the dismemberment of the fetus is that "before it has exited into the atmosphere [that is, where it begins to breathe] it is not a life [*l'av nefesh*] and it may be killed to save its mother."[112] From this statement it is inferred that the fetus (and all the more so an embryo) has no human status and may be disposed of at will. This inference, however, is much too hasty. In fact, Rashi limits this definition of life to the Talmud's discussion of the fetus whose existence directly threatens the life of its mother.

Before we draw any practical inferences from this text or any similar text, we need to note that four terms are used to designate human life: human being (*adam*), fetus (*vlad*), life (*hayyim*), and breathing being (*nefesh*). The first of these words is *adam*, meaning human being. We have learned from one rabbinic text that the unborn child at any stage of its development is considered to be human. Like all such restrictions incumbent upon non-Jews, according to the Talmud this restriction also is incumbent upon Jews. Jewish morality is never less strict, especially regarding human life issues, than non-Jewish morality.[113]

The second word is *vlad* (fetus), which comes from the verb *yalod*, meaning "to be born." Thus, even though the fetus, in utero, is not yet the fully separate being it will be after completing the birth process extra utero, it is called a child in the sense that it is meant to be a child, unless some internal or external factor interferes with its natural end—which is to be born and develop into adulthood. Thus, people who refer to the fetus as an "unborn child" have rabbinic precedent on their side.[114]

The third word designating human life is *hayyim*, the word for life in general. This word is predicated not only of animals but also of God (however metaphorically). In the foregoing text, both the mother and the fetus have life (*hayyim*). Therefore, the issue is not that one is alive and the other (for all intents) is dead; the question is whose life takes precedence in our rescue efforts when only one of them can be saved. The situation might be compared to two people in a well who need to be saved. By saving the one closest to us, we might push the other one down further, in effect drowning the second person. At least we have saved the most proximate life, however.[115]

To add a personal example, this is exactly what I was told happened to my great-grandmother, Jennie Eller. On February 22, 1905, in Chicago, she was about to give birth to her ninth child. Because the baby was too big for her birth canal, it was dismembered in utero to save her life. (She lived until 1943.) Undoubtedly this technique was accepted medical practice even one hundred years ago.[116] It also is what Jewish law mandates be done, and it is eminently rational. I might add, however, that with the prevalence of Caesarian section surgery and with even minimal prenatal care, the need to abort a fetus rather than removing it live from the uterus surgically is rarely required anymore. Furthermore, any woman who has enough access to an abortion clinic has even more access to minimal prenatal care. In other words, this kind of abortion has almost never been a moral option for at least the past fifty or more years in countries such as Canada and the United States.

The fourth word used to designate human life is *nefesh*, which is frequently translated as "soul." This translation is misleading, however. As a result of the influence of the dualistic anthropology of Plato and his philosophical followers, including several significant medieval Jewish theologians, "soul" is taken to be a separate, immortal substance that is temporarily housed within a mortal human body.[117] In biblical anthropology, however, *nefesh* means the ability of organisms to move themselves. All living animals have the status of *nefesh*; plants do not.[118] Therefore, when Rashi states that the fetus in utero is not a *nefesh*, he seems to mean that the fetus that is not yet breathing is in some respects a lesser life than that of his or her mother. The mother is the fetus's enclosing environment; its own movement is not yet part of a separate environment. The fetus is still—literally rooted in its mother's body.[119] Nevertheless, Rashi states explicitly that this analysis is of practical significance only when the fetus is a direct threat to the life of his or her mother, when the principle that "her life takes precedence" (*shehayyeha qodmin*) is enunciated. This situation is akin to amputation of a gangrenous organ or limb, which if not excised will kill its host organism.[120] In no way is Rashi even implying that this principle applies in any other context.[121]

Designating the fetus as not a *nefesh* could be influenced by the following text: "Even an infant [*tinoq*] in his or her first day [extra utero] . . . whoever kills it is liable [for murder]."[122] The Talmud finds the scriptural basis for this ruling in the words, "When a man kills any human life [*nefesh*] whomsoever" (Leviticus 24:17).[123] This analysis, however, simply means that abortion is not considered to be the equivalent of infanticide with regard to capital punishment.[124] Indeed, one can see this dispensation from capital punishment as part of the overall rabbinic trend to restrict capital punishment as much as possible within the limits of the law. Surely that trend is motivated by the same concern that motivates the strict law pertaining to abortion: reverence for the sanctity of human life—even the human life of someone who has committed a sin but could be convicted of less than a capital offense. In all cases, then, the principle of the sanctity of human life should motivate us in all our legal judgments to avoid killing whenever there is even the slightest doubt.[125]

There seems to be a contradiction, however, between the first rabbinic text and the second rabbinic text. The first text seems to make the prohibition of abortion absolute, without any exceptions. The second text clearly makes an exception when the fetus directly threatens the life of his or her mother. Moreover, the first text is made to apply to Noahides—to all humankind—whereas the second text seems to apply only to Jews. Is there a difference in the prohibition of abortion—a stricter one for non-Jews and a more lenient one for Jews? To say that, however, would contravene the talmudic principle: "Nothing permitted to the Jews is forbidden to the non-Jews."[126] As we have seen in the more philosophical treatment of Noahide law, that law is taken up into Mosaic law, giving it a new covenantal status; it also is supplemented by new aspects of Mosaic law. Nonetheless, Noahide law is not fundamentally changed by Mosaic law. It remains obligatory for non-Jews and is literally reiterated in Mosaic law for Jews. The Noahide prohibition of bloodshed (*shefikhut damim*) is reiterated in the Mosaic prohibition "thou shalt not murder" (Exodus 20:13; Deuteronomy 5:17). Accordingly, the prohibition of bloodshed should be identical for Jews and non-Jews.

To resolve this contradiction between Jewish and Noahide law, one could move in two different directions. One could say that because Jewish law is meant to be stricter or at least as strict as Noahide law, Jewish law should not recognize any exceptions to the prohibition of abortion, just as Noahide law seems to recognize no such exceptions. Accordingly, the fetus's right to life should always take precedence. Conversely, one could say that because Jewish law permits or even mandates abortion in cases of a mortal threat to the life of the mother, non-Jewish law ought not be any stricter than Jewish law. Thus, Noahide law should be at least as lenient as Jewish law. Accordingly, the mother's right to life should always take precedence. The question is what *stricter* means: stricter for whom? For whose life are we to be stricter? If we are to be stricter for the sake of the life of the fetus, Jewish law—like (what seems to be) Noahide law—should relinquish the exception when the fetus threatens the life of his or her mother. If we are to be stricter for the sake of the life of the mother, however, Noahide law should relinquish the absolute status it seems to give to the prohibition of abortion. To answer this question, an anonymous medieval comment suggests that the Noahide law should be made to conform to the leniency of the Jewish law regarding abortion, which means that we are to be stricter for the sake of the life of the mother—that her right to life in this situation of mortal conflict trumps the life of the fetus.[127] No reason for this concession is given there, however. For that we must go back to the Talmud.

The text regarding the need for feticide in the case of the fetus that is too big for the birth canal of its mother, which would kill the mother if it were not dismembered before its actual birth, relates to a case brought into a discussion of the law of the pursuer (*rodef*). This law is based on the rationally justifiable warrant for self-defense: "If someone comes to kill you, kill him first" (*hashkem le-horgo*).[128] This mandate is extended to a third party, who is required to save a would-be murder victim (*nirdaf*) from his or her assailant. When the only way to do that is to kill the assailant, the rescuer is mandated to kill that assailant on behalf of the would-be victim. At that point, the blood of the would-be victim is "redder" than the blood of the assailant; in this case, the assailant has waived the sanctity of his or her life.[129] Would-be murderers have forfeited their right to life. This conclusion undoubtedly is based on the rationally justifiable scriptural norm, "Do not stand idly by the blood of your neighbor" (Leviticus 19:16), and on the equally rationally evident rabbinic norm, "One is to benefit another [*zakhin l'adam*] even without his [or her] consent."[130] The latter norm is especially germane in a case of a life-saving abortion inasmuch as the mother rarely, if ever, can act on her own behalf.

The question is whether the would-be murderer or pursuer (*rodef*) needs to be a person whose pursuit of the would-be victim or "the pursued" (*nirdaf*) is acting out of free choice. In other words, to qualify for the status of a pursuer—whom either the pursued or a third party acting on his or her behalf may kill—does this pursuer have to be a sane adult (possessing *mens rea*) or not? Could the pursuer be a child who is below the age of consent? Could the pursuer be a fetus? The Talmud's answer, in two different discussions of the issue, is that defense of the would-be victim is incumbent on anyone regardless of what or who is threatening that life.[131] In this case, one is not required to respect the human life of the pursuer, even if that threat is internal rather than external. The requirement obtains even if that pursuer is neither a free agent nor even a conscious one.

Killing the threatening fetus, notwithstanding its human status, is an unintended consequence of the mother's attempt to save her own life. It is not her direct intention to kill anyone. Nevertheless, the question becomes more complicated when we are dealing with a third-party rescuer, as would almost always be the case in abortion because no women in labor or in any stage of threatening pregnancy are able to operate on themselves. A famous case in the Talmud is germane in this context.

The story is told of two men in the desert; one of them has a flask of water, but there is only enough water for him to survive long enough to reach an inhabited place.[132] Should he drink the water and survive, at the expense of his unfortunate colleague? Should he share the water with his colleague and thus die together with him in the desert? The latter view is that of Ben Petura, who argues that "it is better [*mutav*] that they both drink and die so that one not have to see the death of his colleague." Ben Petura's meaning might be what we call today survivor's guilt, in which one wonders whether it would have been better to have died guiltless with one's fellows than live with the haunting idea that the others really deserved to live more than one did. This attitude is very common among survivors of the Holocaust—some of whom have said things like, "I saved my own life when I could have stayed together with my father and died with him; yet my father was a much better person than I was, am, or ever will be. I feel like I abandoned him." Only a very insensitive fool would attempt to argue with a survivor that his or her feelings of guilt are irrational.

Rabbi Akivah, however, takes the opposite view. Quoting the scriptural verse "your brother shall live with you [*immakh*]" (Leviticus 25:36), he reasons, "Your life takes precedence [*qodmim*] over that of your colleague." Yet one can also see Rabbi Akivah's view as essentially a reasoned opinion (*sevara*) that is based on the evident norm of self-defense.[133] There also is the talmudic principle that "a person is his own closest relative."[134] This principle is invoked as a reason for the inadmissibility of self-incrimination.[135] Citing it in the present context is appropriate for the following reason: Just as one may not incriminate oneself because there is insufficient distance between the witness and the criminal, one must save the one closest to oneself because there is sufficient proximity of the rescuer to the one in mortal danger to be the first one to do so.[136] In cases involving testimony, proximity disqualifies a witness; in cases involving rescue, proximity warrants the most proximate rescuer to rescue a would-be victim, even when that victim is the same person as the rescuer.

The foregoing is the moral dynamic of a two-party relationship, which is like the case in which the pursued is morally enabled to save himself or herself by whatever means necessary, even if it entails a lethal consequence for the other by default. (On the other hand, one is forbidden to actively kill someone else to save one's own life, even if ordered to do so by a powerful third party who has the power to kill one if one does not follow the command to kill another.)[137] The dynamic becomes more complicated, however, when a third party is added—that is, when A is required to rescue B from C. This third-party dynamic arises in the text regarding the woman in hard labor: "But if most of it [the fetus] already exited, then nothing is to be done to it [*ein nog'in bo*]."[138] Recall also that the reason for this proscription is that "one life [*nefesh*] is not to be set aside for another life."

We must now ask: If the fetus in utero is the "pursuer" (albeit an unconscious and nonwilling pursuer) of its mother, why is the newborn infant—who is not even completely extra utero and who is no more conscious than when it was in utero—no longer its mother's pursuer (*rodef*)? In fact, we now see this is what is involved in the issue of "partial birth abortion."

The Babylonian Talmud simply implies that the difference between the fetus in utero and the infant who is even partially extra utero depends on who is the pursuer. The fetus in utero is taken to be the pursuer of its mother, from whom she is to be rescued by a third party who is capable of doing so. But the infant, even when it is still partially in utero, is not taken to be its mother's pursuer. The text offers a very enigmatic explanation of this difference: "There, it is from Heaven [*de-me-shamaya*] that she is being pursued."[139] Undoubtedly on the basis of the fact that the rabbis frequently use the word "Heaven" to denote God's natural (as distinct from God's supernatural or miraculous) causality in the world, Maimonides writes that "this is the nature of the world" (*zehu tiv'o shel olam*).[140] Yet why is this situation any more "natural" than when the mother and her fetus are locked together in a mortal struggle? Moreover, even if the situation is more natural, why are we forbidden to interfere in this natural struggle? If someone were about to be attacked by a wild animal, which is surely natural ("the law of the jungle"), would we not interfere in this natural event?[141]

A better answer to our dilemma might be found in the treatment of this case in the Palestinian Talmud: "Rabbi Boon said in the name of Rav Hisda that it is different there since we do not know who is killing whom [*mi horeg et mi*]."[142] Again, however, why is the fetus in utero more of a pursuer of its mother than the partially exited baby is a pursuer of his or her mother? What is the difference between these two situations?

Surely the difference is one of proximity to the rescuer. In the case of the fetus in utero, the mother as the would-be victim is always more proximate to the external rescuer than the fetus that is still within her body. In the case of the baby who has partially exited from the womb, however, both the baby and the mother are equally proximate to the rescuer. Neither is privileged over the other by virtue of greater proximity versus greater distance. They are equidistant relative to the observer or rescuer. As such, as in all such cases of doubt, the matter is left to the two equal parties to work out for themselves—or, as Maimonides might have said, "Let nature here take its own course." For example, suppose I see A, who is holding a gun, chasing B. I am obligated to save B from A, even though B might also be pursuing A. Nevertheless, as long as I only see A as the pursuer of B, I am obligated to save B's life, even at A's expense, if necessary. If both would-be victims/pursuers are equidistant from me, however, I am obliged, in the words of a talmudic phrase, "to sit and do nothing" (*shev v'al ta'aseh*).[143] If I were to interfere in this case of equidistance, my action in favor of one party, which would necessarily be an action against the other party, would not be based on any rational criterion. It could only be either purely arbitrary (like flipping a coin) or prejudiced (I like A better than I like B).

THE EMBRYO BEFORE AND AFTER
THE FORTIETH DAY OF GESTATION

With regard to embryonic stem cell research, even some traditionalist Jewish ethicists are convinced that just as the life of the fetus ought to be sacrificed when it threatens the life of its mother, the life of the embryo may be—even ought to be—sacrificed to save somebody else's life. Clearly this conclusion would violate the basic principle that "one life is not set aside for another"—that is, if one assumes that the embryo is a person who is the bearer of rights, even if only the most basic right not to be killed. Furthermore, it would violate the sole permission of abortion to the situation in which the fetus (or even the embryo) is a direct threat to the life of its host mother. The question yet to be answered is this: When does human life really begin? If human life in utero is not yet human but only potentially human, it might have no more human status than male sperm or female ova, which also are potentially human—that is, they can be synthesized into a real human being by an act of sexual congress (or in vitro fertilization). When does that conceiving synthesis occur? Precisely when does the fertilization of the female ovum by male sperm become a distinct life of its own, even though it is attached to its mother's body until its actual birth?

To get around the prohibition of abortion altogether, even some traditionalist Jewish ethicists have invoked a talmudic distinction between fetal life before the fortieth day of gestation and after the fortieth day of gestation.[144] Whereas the creation of the embryo (*beri'at ha'ubar*) takes places at the moment of conception, the initial formation of the embryo (*yetsirat ha'vlad*) does not take place until the forty-first day of gestation.[145] The Talmud presents the following imagined scenario: "Rav Judah said in the name of Rav [his teacher] that forty days before the formation of the fetus a heavenly voice goes forth to proclaim: The daughter of X is destined [to be married] to Y."[146] Thus, talmudic sages not only assumed that "marriages are made in heaven" but that we can know exactly when the marriage of that future couple has been predestined. That statement might represent the feeling of happily married people that they were destined for each other even before their respective births—that their marriage was made in heaven.[147] To be sure, such a statement is part of the nonnormative side of Jewish theology (*aggadah*). Nevertheless, such ideas have informed normative (halakhic) judgments.[148] Indeed, the theological assertion that human life begins at conception (*me-sh'at peqidah*) also has halakhic value inasmuch as it indicates that a fetal life has human status even before its formation (*me-sh'at ha-yetsirah*) at forty days.[149]

We can see this idea at work when the Talmud assumes that an embryo that is less than forty days old does not yet seem to have any true human status. Today one might say that it is mere protoplasm. The *locus classicus* in the Talmud states, "The daughter of an Aaronide priest [*bat kohen*] married to an ordinary Jew [*yisrael*] who died. . . . Rav Hisda said that she may immerse herself and eat from [her father's] priestly portion [*terumah*] until forty days [after her Israelite husband's] death."[150] At this point, after the ruling has been stated, the editors of the Talmud give the following explanation: "If she is not pregnant, she is not pregnant; but even if she is pregnant, it [the embryo] is mere water [*maya b'alma*]."[151] Here the law is that the daughter of a priest who is married to a non-priestly Jew who then dies still has the priestly privileges of her father's house until it is evident that she is pregnant with her dead husband's child. Her pregnancy does not have any real consequences for her life, however, until it is more than forty days old. (If her husband had not died, however, and she was still living with him and having intercourse with him, she then loses the priestly privileges of her premarital youth at the time they begin living together as husband and wife, the assumption being that she might very well be pregnant with his child already and that, like most pregnancies, it will be viable to term.)

Here we see an ancient notion that the embryo receives its form at a certain point in its development and that before that time it is inchoate matter.[152] (Note that no biblical verse or specifically Jewish tradition is put forth as the basis of what we can now call the "mere water" principle.) This notion clearly uses the concepts of matter and form that were put forth most influentially in Aristotelian biology. Many ethicists, from late antiquity until the time when microscopic embryonic matter could be discerned, held that the full form of the child is contained in the male's sperm and that after the fortieth day after its insertion into the woman's vagina leading into her uterus it becomes implanted there.[153] This biology seems to have had very wide acceptance in the world of late antiquity in which the discussions of the Talmud took place. As in many other matters, the rabbis no doubt were reiterating generally accepted scientific opinion. The same differentiation (using different scientific distinctions to be sure) is evident in the formal distinction some secularist ethicists have made between human *being* and human *personhood*—a distinction they use to practically differentiate between the life claims of prenatal human life at different stages of intrauterine development and even postuterine development.[154] This interuterine differentiation (i.e., the attempt to differentiate an embryo from a fetus) is spurious with regard to life-or-death questions. The only human being who is not a human person is a corpse, whose human right to decent burial is not a right any living human person could justifiably exercise.[155]

Because we are now told that embryonic cell research is most successfully conducted when the embryo is in its first week, some Jewish ethicists have expanded the "mere water" principle to apply it to the question of killing preembryonic life. These ethicists conclude that an embryo is without the protection of the right to life. Moreover, although some of these same Jewish ethicists are opposed to elective abortion or abortion on demand, they would argue that there is a difference between an abortion to save another human life and an abortion for reasons other than saving another human life. My disagreement with that argument is that the classical Jewish sources that deal with abortion permit it only when a fetus (or even an embryo) is a mortal pursuer of his or her own mother's life when the fetus or embryo is in utero. Surely an embryo that was never in its mother's womb (that is, the womb of the woman from whose egg it was fertilized) could hardly be a threat to that woman's life—or to anyone's life. Nevertheless, these ethicists insist that an embryonic life before its fortieth day of gestation may—some even say must—be used as a means to save *any other* human life. This line of argument is their justification for the use of a week-old embryo for the sole purpose of deriving pluripotent stem cells from it, through a procedure that kills the embryo. Add to this argument the commandment "you shall not stand idly by when your neighbor's life is in peril" (Leviticus 19:16), which is the obligation to save someone else's life, and there seems to be a moral obligation to engage in stem cell research.[156]

That is how the argument goes, if I understand it correctly. Consider, however, the classical Jewish sources that are taken to be the textual basis for this argument. How rational is the argument? How accurate is the interpretation of the talmudic text being used in this argument?

Rashi uses the notion that the forty-day-old or younger embryo is "mere water," to which the Talmud has given the stamp of approval, in three other related contexts.[157] In the laws of inheritance, if an embryo dies before the fortieth day of gestation, a new male fetus conceived after the death of this embryo would be considered the firstborn (*bekhor*) at birth and would, according to biblical law, inherit a share of his father's estate that is twice the amount (*pi shnayim*) inherited by any of his brothers (according to Deuteronomy 21:17). On the other hand, if a fetus died after the fortieth day of gestation, then no fetus conceived after his death would ever have the status of a firstborn child at birth. Rashi says this is because the embryo that is younger than forty days old is "mere water."[158] Moreover, if an embryo that was the first such child conceived by its mother is miscarried before the fortieth day of gestation, a male child conceived subsequently, born, and surviving to his thirtieth day after birth would be the firstborn of his mother. This second child would have to go through the rite of the "redemption of the firstborn son" (*pidyon ha-ben*) prescribed in scripture (Exodus 13:2; Numbers 18:15–16), whereby the father of the real firstborn son is required to given an Aaronide priest (*kohen*) five shekels (or what is taken to be its equivalent in the coin of the realm). Again, the reason for the differentiation is that the embryo before the fortieth day of gestation is "mere water."[159] When the Temple was still in operation (as when it will be in operation again), a woman who miscarried before the fortieth day of her pregnancy would not be considered impure (*tme'ah*) and unfit to enter the Temple precincts until she brought the prescribed sacrifice (Leviticus 12:1–8). Again, Rashi writes that the miscarried fetus is "mere water."[160]

On the basis of these three cases in which Rashi opines that the reason for the rulings is because the fetus is "mere water," some scholars make an inference that entails applying a principle used in one area of law to another area of law. The inference is erroneous, however. Although in all three cases the fetus that is less than forty days old counts for nothing, that assessment obtains only *ex post facto;* hence, one may not infer from this retrospective judgment a prospective warrant (or even permission) to abort this same fetus *ab initio.*[161] Nevertheless, that implication has been drawn and still is being drawn by some traditionalist Jewish ethicists, whose reasoning (but not whose good intentions) I am calling into question.

Erroneous inferences have been made from the "mere water" texts because certain distinctions in talmudic jurisprudential logic have been overlooked. We have two different genres of cases involving conflicting claims, each entailing the hard question of the human status of an embryo before the fortieth day of gestation. The practical questions are as follows: May the daughter of an Aaronide priest who was married to a nonpriestly Jew who has died continue to eat from her father's priestly portion if she miscarried before the fortieth day of her pregnancy? May a son born after the miscarriage of an embryo before the fortieth day of gestation inherit a double portion of his father's estate, or is he no different from the rest of his younger brothers? Should the father of a child born after a miscarriage during the first forty days of gestation redeem a son conceived and born thereafter, or may he claim that his firstborn son has already died and thus refuse to pay the redemption money? May a woman who has miscarried before the fortieth day of pregnancy refuse to buy and bring a sacrifice to the Temple after her miscarriage before forty days, or may the Temple priests insist that she do so? May this pre-forty-day embryo be aborted at will, or does it have enough humanity to foreclose its being killed even to save another human life? Closely related to this last question is the following question: Should this embryo be aborted if the stem cells derived from it will save another human life, or should its own life be saved? There are two different types of conflict involved in these cases.

In the first four cases, there is a conflict of economic interests (*mamonot*). In such cases the burden of proof (*ha-ray'ah*) is on the accuser.[162] In the first case, the young widow who wants to continue to eat from her father's portion would have to prove that she miscarried before the fortieth day of her pregnancy, even if previous assumptions had been otherwise. There is a potential conflict with her other siblings, who might claim that the widow's return to her father's table would diminish the portion they could receive if she had already permanently left her father's table. In the second case, the younger brothers would have to prove that their eldest brother is not really the firstborn son with regard to the right of the firstborn son to a double portion of their late father's estate. They would have to prove that their mother really miscarried after the fortieth day of her pregnancy before the birth of their eldest brother rather than beforehand, even if previously it had been assumed (*hazaqah*) otherwise.[163] They might want to prove this point because their respective shares of their father's estate would increase if their eldest brother were not the real firstborn son (*bekhor*). In the third case, the Aaronide priest, who is entitled to the redemption money for the firstborn son, would have to prove that the mother of this boy miscarried before the fortieth day of a previous pregnancy and that therefore this boy is the firstborn for purposes of redemption, even if it were previously assumed otherwise.[164] Indeed, most priests would want to prove that this child is the firstborn son (*bekhor*) so they could get the redemption money to which they are usually entitled.[165] In the fourth case, the Temple priests would have to prove that the woman who has given birth to her first child miscarried before the fortieth day during her first pregnancy and, therefore, that she owes the Temple a sacrifice because her child is the firstborn for these purposes, even if it were previously assumed otherwise. Indeed, they probably would want to do this so they could eat the portion of the sacrifice brought after childbirth to which they are usually entitled.[166]

In these kinds of cases, the question of when human life begins has to be answered to resolve a monetary conflict. Although these kinds of monetary conflicts also involve specifically Jewish rituals, they should be resolved by the same criteria that are used to resolve ordinary monetary disputes that do not involve any ritual factors.

The tradition establishes a criterion of factual differentiation—forty days of gestation—that seems arbitrary. We might say, however, that the forty-day criterion, which was not unique to Jews, might be based on an empirical factor.[167] That is, by the fortieth day of pregnancy (so I have been told by my wife and other women), most women are already experiencing the symptoms of pregnancy such as a missed menstrual period and nausea (morning sickness). Before that time, a woman could miscarry and not even be aware of the fact that she had been pregnant. She might think that the miscarriage is either a late menstrual discharge or some sort of abnormal vaginal bleeding, especially in the era when gynecology was not yet a medical discipline and women could not get the type of gynecological diagnosis they can get today.[168]

In the fifth and sixth cases, however, which involve the question of killing the embryo before the fortieth day of gestation, we have a conflict of lives. We are being asked to allow one life to be killed so that another one *might* live. The case is even stronger if we are asked to allow one life to be killed because another life *should* live. In any question of conflict involving lives (*nefashot*), the law is in favor of the most proximate life, as we have seen. The human right to life always trumps any other right. That is so even when the right to life is certain (*bari*) and the right to a possible cure of even fatal deformities is still doubtful (*shema*).[169] This overall question became a hotly debated question in the 1970s when heart transplant operations were becoming accepted medical procedure. There was a question about whether some of the heart donors were really dead before their donation was given to *potentially* save the life of someone with a badly damaged heart by replacing it with their own.

Unlike the first four cases, which deal with conflicts of economic interests, in cases in which there is a human life to be saved, that life need not prove—that is, have proved on his or her behalf—anything to make its vital claim on us. Its nonhuman existence must be proved by someone else who wants to use it instrumentally. In this context, however, the best criterion for determining when human life begins should be what is less disputable than its rivals. That least disputable time for determining the beginning of human life is the moment of conception. It could not be a unique human life before conception because it does not have its own DNA; it could only be a human life upon its conception when it does have its own DNA.[170] This determination helps to resolve any conflict even between an embryo's right to life and a fully developed person's right to life-saving medical treatment. We are to act in favor of actual human life over the probability of saving or enhancing another human life.

The presumption in favor of actual human life also obtains in a case of conflict between a person and the law when human life is at stake (*piquah nefesh*). Thus, if there is a conflict regarding whether to save a human life through violation of the Sabbath law or to keep the Sabbath law and thereby sacrifice, or even endanger, a human life, the conflict is resolved by violating the Sabbath law to save the human life.[171] Furthermore, if there is doubt about whether the person for whom we are violating the Sabbath is even still alive, we still resolve that doubt in favor of that person. (The case given in the Talmud involves a person buried under rubble on the Sabbath; we will not know whether he or she is alive until after we have violated the Sabbath by digging the body out from under the rubble.)[172] Along these lines, the great medieval jurist and theologian Nahmanides rules that one should even violate the Sabbath or Yom Kippur to save a fetus that is less than forty days old.[173]

Conversely, however, in a conflict between a person and the law in which human life is not at stake, the conflict is resolved in favor of the law. Thus, if there is a conflict regarding whether to earn a living through violation of the Sabbath law or to keep the Sabbath law and thereby endanger one's livelihood, the conflict is resolved in favor of the Sabbath law, even if that choice entails economic loss.[174]

Finally, even if one holds that a fetus that is less than forty-one days old is "mere water"—meaning that its demise has no legal consequences—we should not infer that actively killing it is permitted. Along these lines, one who kills a person who was already mortally wounded (*treifah*) is exempt from capital punishment by a human court because we cannot ascertain what (or who) was the actual cause of death. Nonetheless, no one could or should infer from this doubtful situation any permission to kill such a person with impunity.[175] Similarly, the fact that a baby is regarded as nonviable at birth does not mean that someone may kill that baby with impunity.[176]

LAW AND SCIENTIFIC EVIDENCE

The principle that states that the embryo before the fortieth day of gestation is "mere water" (*maya b'alma*) should not be applied to the question of whether one may kill such an embryo, even if stem cells derived from the embryo might be used in medical procedures that might save the lives of other humans. Yet there are some Jewish ethicists, even of a traditionalist bent, who have taken this principle as their basis for permitting or even warranting the lethal procedure of deriving stem cells from living embryos that are less than forty days old.

We now need to look into the logic used in the formulation of the "mere water" principle. Is it a legal fiat? Have the rabbis simply stipulated in an apodictic way a boundary between life that has the protection of law and fetal life that lacks that protection? If that is what this principle is, it cannot be applied to cases in which the rabbis themselves did not explicitly apply it or it is obviously assumed to operate. Furthermore, one may doubt whether "mere water" is really a principle at all in the talmudic sense. In fact, it is not called a principle (*kelal* in Hebrew, *klala* in Aramaic) in the Talmud or by Rashi. As such, "mere water" functions only as a generalization, given as a reason for a particular legal ruling long after that particular ruling had already been made. A true principle, however, functions both as a general explanation for a ruling already made and as a generalization that can be the inclusive basis of new rulings not yet made.[177] The fact that "mere water" is not designated as a principle means that it is to be applied only where it has already been applied—and nowhere else. There is no evidence in either the talmudic sources or the medieval (*rish'onim*) representations of them that "mere water" was ever taken to be an inclusive generalization. "Mere water," then, functions heuristically, not constructively.

What if the "mere water" explanation is not a legal fiat, however, but a scientific opinion? Unlike a legal fiat, any such scientific judgment is open to the following question: Is it true or not? That is, does this scientific opinion correspond to the phenomenon it bespeaks or not? As a statement of fact rather than a legal fiat, the assertion that an embryo that is less than forty days old is "mere water" cannot escape having its truth value validated or invalidated. A legal fiat, conversely, can be questioned only with regard to whether it is coherent. It can be questioned only with regard to its meaning, not its scientific truth value.

As a scientific opinion, "mere water" could more easily be used constructively in new cases to which it has not previously been applied. As such, anyone who wishes to use the "mere water" opinion to justify killing an embryo because it is "mere water" will have to be prepared to subject it to scientific scrutiny. There is always the chance that newer and better science will show an earlier scientific explanation to be false. Thus, the constructive possibility of "mere water" as a scientific opinion is greater, but so is its vulnerability in that it could be overruled in the court of scientific inquiry. If it were only a legal fiat, it could not be overruled by science; as we have seen, however, as a legal fiat the principle can be applied only to explain old law, not construct new law.

Current scientific opinion certainly would not regard the embryo as lacking its own unique human properties until the fortieth day of gestation. Therefore, however well-intentioned (what distinguishes an error from a lie, a mistake from deceit) the rabbis who judged the embryo to be "mere water" before the fortieth day of gestation were, current scientific opinion would have to say they erred. They erred because they did not have the scientific means we now have for obtaining evidence about what is actually occurring in embryonic life from its very conception. The accepted fact now is that from the moment of conception the embryo has its own DNA, it own unique genetic code.

This fact (which is more than mere hypothesis) raises what seems to be the great irony in the position of ethicists who want to use the "mere water" criterion to justify killing an embryo to derive its pluripotent stem cells. How can an embryo's stem cells have any medical value if they are "mere water"? Advocates who would use stem cells taken from live embryos to save other human lives would do so only if they were convinced scientifically that these live embryos have uniquely human properties that are valuable because they are able to create healthy tissue in diseased human bodies. Use of these pluripotent stem cells might save those diseased human bodies from dying of their present diseases. Yet does the necessary killing of the embryo from which they have been taken not involve killing a uniquely human life? By "uniquely human life" I mean that as a member of the unique human species, this life has human DNA genetically, and it has its own particular variety of human DNA as a unique individual. Is using scientific evidence so arbitrarily in one's moral judgments not irrational? Such arbitrariness seems to be both bad theology and bad philosophy. It is bad theology when it is used to make a legal judgment for Jews, and it is worse philosophy when it enters the type of secular public discussion that at its best must use truly universal categories and principles.

This answer is enough for philosophy. The "mere water" principle or explanation has no philosophical value because it has no scientific value. Philosophically speaking, one could say that we do not derive an *ought* from an *is*. Nevertheless, we do derive an *is* from an *ought*—not in the strict logical sense of inference but in the sense that our concern with any factual matter (any *is*) stems from our prior concern with the question of what we are to do or not do with it. In the case before us, our first concern is with the *ought* question: What may we or should we do with this embryo to which we now have technological access? (I say "we" rather than "I" because as with any technological procedure, the procedure always involves a cooperative rather than solo effort.) To answer that question intelligently, however, we need to discover and ascertain by the most current scientific criteria what this embryo is. If it is human per se, we may not/should not harm it in any way. If it is not human, then some justifiable purpose—such as possibly saving the human life of another person—might justify our doing anything with that embryo that the fulfillment of this justifiable purpose requires.

The philosophical use of natural science is teleological: science pursued for the sake of a prior normative end. Nevertheless, the teleology is moral, which means that it is not inherent in the subject matter of that science itself when it functions autonomously in it own realm. As such, philosophy can use scientifically ascertained data for its own purposes, and these purposes make moral claims upon us—as Kant well understood when he reserved the German word for "end" or *telos*—*Zweck*—for persons rather than for things or even states of affairs.[178] Philosophy may use scientifically obtained information only for the sake of its own purposes; however, it may not alter or distort what it has taken from science. Philosophy should take only what science, as it were, gives it intact. The same applies for theology (which, as we have seen, also must be careful to take what philosophy gives it intact and not distort it). Thus, both philosophy and theology say more than the scientific data they use in their normative propositions, but they may not make scientifically ascertained facts say something essentially different from what they say in their own scientific realm.

Furthermore, theology has a problem of its own that it does not share with philosophy. The problem pertains to the four strictly theological or ritual questions (remember that Jewish law/*halakhah* is the practical side of Jewish theology) to which the "mere water" principle has been applied. The problematic question is the following: If the "mere water" principle that is used to explain the law in these four cases is meant to be a scientific opinion, what happens when that scientific opinion is proven to be false? Should these laws be changed as a result of our newer and seemingly better scientific information about prenatal development? Moreover, is there any difference between cases involving human life and cases that do not involve life with regard to the use or disuse of scientific facts?

In the cases in which the fetus has no status during the first forty days of gestation, all the normative questions are uniquely Jewish. These four cases deal with four highly specialized matters of Jewish ritual law. Moreover, even though there are economic considerations, these considerations all have direct ritual consequences. We are not dealing with property in the ordinary sense, nor are we dealing with stages of human life affecting property rights in the ordinary sense. As such, special categories obtain; conversely, the categories used in reasoning about universal moral questions also do not fully obtain.

For Jews, universal moral questions pertain to Noahide law. That is especially so when Noahide law is regarded as the Jewish name for natural law. Noahide law is of concern to Jews when they are involved with non-Jews in a common moral realm (such as the secular societies in which most Jews now live) or when Jews are looking for the normative preconditions for what subsequently became Jewish law—preconditions that still influence the way Jewish law is interpreted in theory and applied in practice. This influence, however, operates only in areas of Jewish law that deal with questions of ordinary human action, such as abortion. Nevertheless, these normative preconditions are rational and thus knowable *a priori*. The universality of Noahide law as natural law is not only about where the law applies (everywhere) and when it applies (in every era); it is especially about how the law is formulated. That formulation is the rationally persuasive representation of or argument for these humanly indispensable norms. Thus, they are binding because they have universal reasons. These laws are binding because no one who accepts his or her human nature and the human nature of all other human persons could have a valid reason to declare them inoperative. Moreover, contrary to Jewish theologians who also are legal positivists, these laws are not binding because of the authority of the Jewish tradition, whether that authority is religious, moral, or political.[179]

Even if some seemingly unique Jewish religious or cultural practices have analogues in other cultures, they are not objects of universal concern; they are only matters of comparative interest. Jews still perform these practices in ways that are uniquely Jewish, phenomenologically speaking. They are of interest only to people who are engaged in comparative cultural studies. There is no real universal moral urgency about them. If these practices have features in common with Jewish practices, they are matters of historical coincidence, even historical influence; these common practices are not matters of universal moral concern. Accordingly, Jews are not required to be concerned with these analogous practices as they are required to be concerned with universally justified practices that have been incorporated virtually intact into their own tradition. The universality of natural law is not the same as historical overlappings studied by comparative religion.

With regard to abortion, however, there is a universal moral question that Jews need to discuss among themselves and among the non-Jews with whom they share common social space. This discussion is necessary because abortion now takes place in public spaces such as hospitals and abortion clinics. Conversely, with regard to issues such as inheritance law and rites of passage such as the redemption of the firstborn son, although there might be analogues in other cultures, they are not issues involving the common social space Jews share with non-Jews or the common moral logic Jews can and should share with non-Jews. Furthermore, the authorized status of these practices in the Jewish tradition comes from sinaitic revelation and the traditional legislation stemming from that revelation, even though there might have been similar practices elsewhere both before and after that revelation to Israel. Therefore, with regard to such special religious practices, Jews need not look for normative sources of these practices in their own prehistory, and they should not proclaim to other cultures that have arisen before or after them in history that Judaism is the normative source of the unique practices of these newer cultures. Such practices are phenomenologically constituted differently in different cultures, however similar they might seem to be superficially. Yet when we address the question of abortion, surely the phenomenon itself is constituted similarly everywhere, and its normative status can best be debated by using universal criteria everywhere.

Even though the four cases in which the "mere water" principle is used as an explanation deal with monetary claims (*mamonot*), they are not ordinary monetary claims. If they were ordinary monetary claims, universal rational standards would apply. In our case, if they were only ordinary monetary claims, the new scientific ascertainment of when human life begins would have to replace the old and inaccurate "mere water" definition. These four cases, however, involve uniquely Jewish phenomena: the priestly gifts (*terumah*), the rights of the firstborn son (*bekhorah*), the redemption of the firstborn son from the priest (*pidyon ha-ben*), and the sacrificial system (*qorbanot*). They have a distinctly ritual (*issura*) character.[180] In such matters, the tradition uses criteria that are stipulated by legal fiat and are not meant to be based on scientific criteria that can be validated or invalidated. That is what makes an issue such as abortion, which deals with a clearly universal human phenomenon, different and thus beholden to different criteria for its interpretation.

In the twelfth century, Maimonides made a fundamental distinction between reasoning on ritual or specifically religious questions and reasoning on general moral questions. This distinction concerns the use of scientific evidence for moral deliberations, which makes it germane to the debate regarding embryonic stem cell research. Maimonides' distinction concerns the difference between using scientific evidence about the imminent mortality of animals, which affects how a Jew is to relate to their being slaughtered for food, and using scientific evidence about the imminent mortality of human beings, which affects how we are to judge acts done to them and by them.

Jews are concerned with the imminent mortality of animals because an animal that is judged to be suffering a mortal lesion (*treifah*) may not be slaughtered for food. It is not kosher.[181] What determines whether the lesion is mortal? Maimonides' answer is that such a determination comes from tradition.[182] What if current scientific opinion tells us, however, that what the tradition has determined to be mortal is based on faulty science? What if, in fact, current science says that what the tradition says is lethal is really vital? What if what the tradition says is vital science now says is really lethal? And what if current science has better evidence for its view than the tradition has for its view?

Maimonides' answer is that scientific evidence (*derekh refu'ah:* literally, "the way of medicine") is irrelevant because we are not dealing with a phenomenon to which universalizable reason (of which scientific research is a part) pertains.[183] Traditional authority is normatively sufficient. The only valid use of scientific evidence in this area would be if scientific evidence enabled us to discover that what we had been permitted to eat is, in fact, dangerous to human life and health. In such a case, the presumption would be in favor of human life, as scientifically understood, over the tradition (*hamira saqanta me'isura*).[184]

Whereas the scientific criterion of viable or nonviable life is of no concern when we are dealing with animals meant for human consumption, it is central in cases involving the imminent mortality of a human being. The question with which Maimonides deals involves a case in which someone has assaulted another person who was suffering from an imminently fatal wound (*terifah*) and died immediately after the assault. Could the assailant be convicted as a murderer? In this case the benefit of the doubt should be in favor of the criminal (*safeq nefashot le-haqel*), who is still a human person, because we cannot be sure whether the victim died because of the act of the human assailant or because of the imminently fatal wound the victim was already bearing.[185]

Who determines whether the earlier wound is fatal or not? To whom do we listen: ancient tradition or contemporary science? Maimonides' answer is that we listen to the scientists (*ha-rof'im:*

literally, "the physicians").[186] Why do we listen to scientific evidence about human life, however, if we do not listen to scientific evidence about animal life? The answer seems to be that, aside from the issue of safety—which animals may be eaten and what condition their meat may be in to be eaten—all that is a specifically Jewish concern. The norms that obtain in our relations with animals at this level are not rational but traditional (*shim'iyot:* "heard," not *sikhliyot:* "reasoned").[187] Human life, on the other hand, is a universal human concern. The norms that obtain are rational norms. They all have evident reasons.[188] Hence, even in inter-Jewish conversations on these matters, the authority of the tradition should not override the exercise of universal human reason.[189] Scientific evidence is an essential component of our larger moral reasoning on all biomedical questions, which now include the issue of embryonic stem cell research.

THE BEGINNING OF HUMAN LIFE

The scientific question is: When does human life begin? One could say that human life begins at birth—namely, when the fetus has fully emerged from his or her mother's body. This position, however, usually is based on seeing human life as a continuum from the *terminus a quo* of birth to the *terminus ad quem* of death. There is a difference, however, between the event of birth and the event of death.

In the event of death, there is no empirical evidence of any personal continuity with what comes after death. (There is only theological evidence for the possibility of life after death in the testimony of sacred texts).[190] Furthermore, even long after anyone would say a person is dead, the dead body still is made up of the same DNA it received at the time of its conception; hence, definitions of death cannot use a scientifically irreducible point of demarcation. Thus, there has to be a designation of a certain point in the history of the human body as an organism that will have to be designated as the *terminus ad quem* of the life of the human person, thereby distinguishing a human person from a human corpse.[191] Just as a human person has the right to live, a human corpse has the right to be buried—or, more accurately, we have the obligation to bury it.[192] In most human traditions, that point of demarcation has been the presence or absence of spontaneous breath.[193]

Regarding the event of birth, however, there is empirical and scientific evidence of personal continuity with what came before birth. Therefore, birth is more of a transition from mediated to immediate human presence in the world than an absolute beginning. A baby does not emerge out of nothing (*ex nihilo*) at its birth, whereas a corpse—as far as we can see, in any case—goes nowhere.[194]

There have been various suggestions about when during prenatal human life we consider human personhood to begin. Some ethicists have suggested that personal beginning is when the fetus develops its own functioning nervous system.[195] There also is the older, more empirical criterion of "quickening"—that is, when the fetus's movement in utero is felt by its mother. All of these suggestions, whether they are scientific or empirical, suffer from a moral dilemma, however: What if human life really begins at an earlier stage? Might not all these distinctions be based on what is not a real difference in kind? Does the lack of such a real difference not indicate a doubtful state of affairs? Don't we have the principle that in cases of doubt we presume in favor of life (*safeq nefashot le-haqel*)?[196] Are not all such doubts dispelled if we assume that human life begins at conception? How could we doubt that there is any beginning we might have missed when we begin at the earliest possible beginning of a distinct human life? We can imagine no earlier beginning than the moment of conception.

In an attempt to push this argument to its irrational extreme (*reductio ad absurdum*), some critics have said that we might as well outlaw destroying sperm or ova as bloodshed. Are they, too, not potential life? Yes, but only in the sense that they have a potential *for* life inasmuch as they have the ability (the potency) to become an embryo—but only when they are brought together in an act they cannot do by themselves for themselves. A sperm and an ovum need to be brought together by someone else, either by an act of normal sexual intercourse between a man and a woman or by the intervention of a scientist in a laboratory. Before they are brought together to procreate something new, their DNA is different from the DNA of this new creature to whose life they have contributed.

The argument for the inviolability of embryonic life is not because it has potential *for* life; it is a human life that already has all the potential, all the unique DNA it needs, for its natural development— unless, of course, someone or something external interferes with the trajectory of that natural development by killing it. When that interference is effected by a thing (e.g., a destructive virus), we regard it as an accident or miscarriage, morally speaking. When this interference is willfully effected by a person, however, we regard it as an abortion, morally speaking.

At this point I would ask my fellow Jewish ethicists, especially the traditionalist ones: Does our reverence for human life as the image of God not require that we treat every human life, even the minuscule human life of the newly conceived embryo, with what the tradition calls "human dignity" (*kvod ha-beriyot*)?[197] Surely we are not obligated or even permitted to kill a human life, however prehuman it now looks, for the sake of somebody else's therapeutic needs—that is, for the sake of somebody to whose life the embryo is not a direct threat. We certainly are not obligated or even permitted to kill an embryo for the more indirect benefit of the advancement of possibly helpful scientific information. I believe that we are neither obligated nor permitted to do so. I believe that we are prohibited from doing so. We can discover that prohibition (*issur*) philosophically and thus argue it to anyone, anywhere, at any time. The argument need not be confined to persons who are required to live according to our own moral theology, although our moral theology certainly can confirm it.

That position is fully consistent with Maimonides' emphasis on how important advances in scientific knowledge are for our moral deliberations about universal human phenomena. Thus, the discovery of DNA and when it first emerges in a human being should change our thinking about the beginning of human life in the same way that the discovery that babies born in the eighth month of pregnancy are viable (*ben qayyama*) changed our thinking about early infant life, even though in the days of the Talmud people believed that they were not viable.[198] Jews are bound by halakhic norms. With regard to questions of human life and death, however, they are not bound to some of their applications that are based on what we now know to have been inaccurate, outdated science. The science of the Talmud has been superseded by more current science, which itself might be superseded in the future. That is why all scientific opinions, even those that attain the status of facts, are tentative. That also is why we have not heard the final word about embryonic stem cells and what we may or may not do with them. Only certain moral or religious truths need to be taken as insuperable. They are either *a priori*, and thus not subject to changing historical conditions, or *a posteriori*, yet unusual in that they come from revelation and not ordinary experience and thus are unchanging because God's word "stands forever" (Isaiah 40:8). Scientific facts, however, fall into neither category.

Yet even Jewish ethicists who see a legal permission (*heter*) for the use of embryonic stem cells for biomedical research intended for life-saving results in the classical Jewish sources cannot make a case that there is an obligation (*hiyyuv*) to do so. The connection between killing the embryo and saving another human life is still much too tenuous. No diseased person for whom scientists hope something emerging from research on embryonic stem cells will save his or her life has enough direct evidence to make a claim on a particular embryo donor of the form, "If you don't turn this embryo over to medical research, you are thereby killing me."

PERMISSION OR OBLIGATION?

Some acts are permitted simply because they have never been forbidden. With regard to stem cells, how could their derivation from live embryos have been explicitly permitted or forbidden by the ancient rabbis when we have just recently learned of their existence, by means of scientific instruments unknown to ancient technology? Nevertheless, there are acts that may be permitted—from the silence of the tradition, as it were—and still ought not be done, even if we now know how to do them where our ancestors did not. (Think of our moral revulsion when some scientists insist that what can be done must be done in cases of their new discoveries and techniques, regardless of the moral problems they involve.) There are several cases in the classical Jewish sources in which the rabbis rule that even though something may be done according to specific legal reasons, it still ought not be done for more general moral reasons.

The best example appears in an important rabbinic responsum written in the seventeenth century by a major German-Jewish jurist, Hayyim Yair Bachrach. In discussing a request for permission for an elective abortion, he notes that one could find several specific legal reasons for such permission (*heter gamur*). He also notes that various distinctions made within fetal life, such as the distinction made between fetal life before and after the fortieth day of gestation, are morally irrelevant in dealing with abortion. Nevertheless, he concludes that elective abortion ought not be permitted because of "the clear practice (*ha-minhag ha-pashut*) that obtains among ourselves and them [the Christians], which is for the sake of public morality." Literally, he refers to a fence (*geder*)— that is, an inhibition—of "rampantly immoral women [*perutsot he-meritsot*] and those men who stray after them."[199] This fence is for the sake of inhibiting irresponsible sexuality. It is based on the concern that if elective abortion were readily permitted, it would make women and men far less responsible for their sexual acts. (Interestingly enough, there seems to be an assumption that ordinary married couples would not want to abort their offspring.) Thus, prohibiting elective abortion is regarded as a deterrent to sexual promiscuity.

The situation is not very different today. Abortion is still largely the recourse of persons who either did not practice birth control or whose birth control device failed them. As such, they want their offspring to be considered their property, which they may either keep or dispose of at will. In other words, they accept no responsibility for the care of the human life their own acts have enabled to come into being—a possibility of which they certainly were aware. Yet such persons often offer the excuse that they never intended to have a child; it was "an accident." Of course, one could say to them that any male–female sexual union must accept responsibility for the ever-present possibility that a child will be the result of their sexual union, even if they practice birth control. If we cannot justify killing the specifically unintended, accidental result of a voluntary sexual encounter between a woman and a man, how much more can we not justify killing the intended result of the voluntary donation of sperm and egg for the conception of an embryo? Even if this embryo is slated to be killed to give its pluripotent stem cells to someone else to save their life, can we use illicit means even for a good end?[200] Indeed, by procreating an embryo for the most immediate purpose, which is to kill it, are we not justifying something far worse than promiscuity? Have we not, in effect, revived human sacrifice and justified it by making it a medical procedure?

Even if we could justify the use of embryonic stem cells for medical research by drawing on the details of Jewish tradition and its specific rules, we need to consider whether such permission is indeed contributing to a moral culture whose purposes are very much at odds with the overall purposes of that religious tradition. Do we want to contribute to a moral culture for which human life, at every stage of its development, is essentially a commodity to be bought and sold, used or discarded, and ultimately the property of whoever has the most power? That is the question any ethicist who posits an irreducible sanctity of human life cannot avoid. Thus, religious ethicists for whom natural law is the necessary minimum and secular ethicists for whom natural law is the optimal maximum both need to examine the legalities of embryonic stem cell research in terms of principles or ends, not just in terms of specific rules.

POLITICAL REALITIES

Given present political realities, a legal ban on embryonic stem cell research is unlikely to be enacted by executive order or legislation. Even if it were enacted, it would be unlikely to pass judicial review—especially in the United States, where the legalization of abortion that came down from the Supreme Court in 1973 in *Roe v. Wade* now seems to have the status of binding precedent (*stare decisis*). The same could be said for the Morgenthaler decision by the Supreme Court of Canada in 1988. Moreover, the legal permissibility of sperm banks and ova banks, where men and women can conceive children anonymously, seems to indicate that there are no legal restraints on any kind of procreation by consenting adults.

Why should anyone attempt to make a political argument for such a ban? Isn't it a matter of moral obscurantism? Isn't it at odds with the whole political, legal, and cultural trajectory of our society? Don't those of us who think lethal embryonic stem cell research ought not be done risk becoming even more politically, legally, and culturally marginalized?

I propose two answers to these questions. First, because most of us who advocate this natural law position are religious, we can hope that our God will influence—in ways mysterious to us—more and more members of our society to demand that respect for the inherent human dignity of all human life, at whatever stage of its development, be consistently affirmed and implemented. This hope is part of our belief that whereas reason can discover the justice that *ought* to be done, only faith leads us to hope that justice *will* be done, sooner or later. Second, we can simply hope that embryonic stem cell research will not deliver the results its proponents have promised us and that we can derive the promised benefits from using sources for stem cell research other than live embryos. Fortunately, not all scientists think that embryos are the only or even the best source of pluripotent stem cells.[201]

If neither of these two answers to our political dilemma occurs, however, and if permission of embryonic stem cell research becomes the law, we will have one more chapter in the continuing movement away from the historical source of most of our moral norms, which is what some call the Judeo-Christian tradition—a key part of which is recognition of natural law. If this movement away from this historical source continues unabated, one might have to make a painful political choice: whether one can remain loyal to a political regime that has moved so far from its cultural sources, especially regarding the respect for human life that characterizes the Judeo-Christian source. Let us hope, therefore, that political revulsion at embryonic stem cell research for what it truly is will lead to political results that could be regarded as a reversal of this overall trajectory. That reversal requires renewed efforts to reeducate the electorate and their representatives. Toward this end, the best course is to formulate the natural law arguments in the most convincing way possible—first to ourselves and then to others. These arguments are inspired by our religious traditions; indeed, they are presupposed by these traditions, although they are not specifically derived from them. Moreover, these natural law arguments can inspire our political process when we make them with conviction and intelligence. Indeed, the faith of most natural law thinkers and doers prevents them from losing hope and helps them appreciate what an ancient rabbi taught: "It is not for you to complete the labor, nor are you free to desist therefrom . . . the Master of your labor can be trusted to bring about the final and everlasting effect of your labor."[202]

NOTES

The following abbreviations for classical Jewish sources are used throughout these notes:

B.   *Babylonian Talmud (Bavli)*

M.   *Mishnah*

MT   *Mishneh Torah* (Maimonides)

T.   *Tosefta*

Tos.   *Tosafot*

Y.   *Palestinian Talmud (Yerushalmi)*

Unless otherwise noted, all translations are by the author.

1. Carina Dennis, "Cloning: Mining the Secrets of the Egg," *Nature* 439 (February 9, 2006): 655. The scientific literature on stem cell research is quite large already. For a good summary of the juncture of science and ethics on this issue, see A. S. Daar and Lorraine Sheremeta, "The Science of Stem Cells: Some Implications for Law and Policy," *Health Law Review* 11 (2003): 5–13.
2. See, e.g., B. Berakhot 26a and Tos., s.v. "ta'ah."
3. See, e.g., M. Arakhin 8.7.
4. See Friedrich Nietzsche, *The Will to Power*, trans. W. Kaufmann and R. J. Hollingdale (New York: Random House, 1967), nos. 141, 298, 471, 552.
5. T. S. Eliot, *Murder in the Cathedral*, pt. 2, in *The Complete Poems and Plays* (New York: Harcourt, Brace, and World, 1971), 220: "Thy glory is declared even in that which denies Thee; the darkness declares the glory of light. Those who deny Thee could not deny, if Thou didst not exist; and their denial is never complete, for if it were so, they would

not exist." In other words, Eliot agrees with Nietzsche that no one is unrelated to God, and then he answers him. The question is only whether one's God is living or dead. Thus, atheism requires theism— if only to deny it—in a way that theism does not require atheism.

6. See David Novak, *Natural Law in Judaism* (Cambridge: Cambridge University Press, 1998), 164–73.

7. See Martin Buber, *I and Thou*, pt. 3, trans. W. Kaufmann (New York: Chas. Scribner's Sons, 1970), 129–30.

8. "Thou" is the now indispensable translation of Buber's *du*, which is the intimate German term for "you"—which can be used only when one is addressing another person or being addressed by another person. The less intimate *Sie*, however, primarily refers to a thing (an "it" or "*es*" in German) and only secondarily to a person. *I and Thou* was the title given to Buber's 1923 masterwork, *Ich und Du*, by its original English translator, Ronald Gregor Smith, in 1937, undoubtedly to show the English reader the uniquely personal meaning of Buber's *du*.

9. Therefore, engaging in willful lying (*sheqer*) is a more serious moral offense than making an erroneous judgment (*ta'ut*). An erroneous judgment is culpable, though less so than willful deceit, only when the exercise of greater care could have prevented the error from having been made in the first place (see, e.g., B. Sanhedrin 33b and Tos., s.v. "she'irvan"). When it is less than that, an erroneous judgment could be termed an "honest mistake." Today, we often hear of scientific hoaxes foisted on the public by unscrupulous scientists. Clearly, their motive for such treachery is to enhance their professional reputation and often their wealth. (Regarding how lies are used for personal profit, see Maimonides, *Commentary on the Mishnah:* Avodah Zarah 4.7.) Indeed, the Talmud calls lying for personal profit *genevat da'at*, "stealing the esteem or the confidence of the person to whom one has lied" (see B. Hullin 94a; Maimonides, MT: Deot, 2.6). Hence, the moral character of a scientist, whether he or she manifests the character trait or virtue of truth-telling or not, will have considerable influence on his or her commitment to the discovery and representation of scientific truth and whether we can believe their claims upon us for acceptance of their scientific conclusions. See Hermann Cohen, *Religion of Reason out of the Sources of Judaism*, trans. S. Kaplan (New York: Frederick Ungar, 1972), 410.

10. For the proper theoretical (*theory* coming from the Greek *theōrein*, "to gaze") appreciation of nature as divine creation, see B. Shabbat 75a regarding Isa. 5:12 and Deut. 4:6; B. Berakhot 43b regarding Eccl.

3:11. For the proper practical appropriation of created nature, see T. Berakhot 4.1 regarding Ps. 24:1 and Prov. 16:4; B. Berakhot 35a–b regarding Prov. 28:4; Y. Berakhot 6.1/9d regarding Deut. 22:9. For discussion of the prohibition of wanton destruction of God's creation, see David Novak, *Jewish Social Ethics* (New York: Oxford University Press, 1992), 118–32.

11. See Immanuel Kant, *Groundwork of the Metaphysic of Morals*, trans. H. J. Paton (New York: Harper, 1964), 59.

12. See David Novak, *The Election of Israel* (Cambridge: Cambridge University Press, 1995), 54–64.

13. See Aristotle, *Nicomachean Ethics*, 1.3/1095a1–10.

14. See B. Shabbat 88a regarding Exod. 19:17.

15. For this logic, see B. Baba Kama 118a.

16. See B. Sanhedrin 72a regarding Exod. 22:1–2. This is the one case where Jewish law seems to mandate punishment in anticipation of a crime yet to be committed (M. Sanhedrin 8.5; *cf.* B. Rosh Hashanah 16b regarding Gen. 21:17). See also *Digest*, 9.2.4pr; 9.2.45.4; 9.2.5. (For these citations, see Bruce Frier, *A Casebook on the Roman Law of Delict* [Atlanta: Scholars Press, 1998], *passim*.)

17. See B. Sanhedrin 72a regarding Exod. 21:2; Maimonides, MT: Rotseah, 1.13 and Joseph Karo, *Kesef Mishneh* thereon.

18. For some of my halakhic responsa, written in my capacity as the coordinator of the Panel of Halakhic Inquiry of the Union for Traditional Judaism, see *Tomeikh KaHalakhah: Responsa of the Panel of Halakhic Inquiry*, ed. W. R. Allen (Teaneck, N.J.: Union for Traditional Judaism, 1994), *passim*. There also are some earlier responsa of mine in David Novak, *Law and Theology in Judaism* I–II (New York, KTAV, 1974–76), *passim*.

19. Aristotle, *Nicomachean Ethics*, 5.1/1129b25-26; see also *Politics*, 1.1/1253a1–20.

20. Hermann Cohen, *Jüdische Schriften*, vol. 3, ed. B. Strauss (Berlin: C. A. Schwetschke und Sohn, 1924), 302.

21. Germain Grisez, "The First Principle of Practical Reason," *Natural Law Forum* 10 (1965): 174.

22. See T. Sheqalim 2.2 regarding Prov. 3:4.

23. See B. Rosh Hashanah 17b.

24. See Maimonides, MT: Mamrim, 1.1–2.

25. See B. Shabbat 23a regarding Deut. 17:1 and 32:7; Y. Sukkah 3.4/53d.

26. *Sifra*: Aharei-Mot, ed. Weiss, 86b, and B. Sanhedrin 59a regarding Lev. 18:5.

27. Se B. Yevamot 47a.

28. See David Novak, "Are Philosophical Proofs of the Existence of God Theologically Meaningful?" in *Talking with Christians* (Grand Rapids, Mich.: Eerdmans Publishing Co., 2005), 247–59.

29. See Baruch Spinoza, *Tractatus Theologico-Politicus*, chap. 17.

30. See Thomas Aquinas, *Summa Theologiae*, 2/1, q. 95, a. 2; q. 96, a. 4 ad 2.

31. See Karl Jaspers, *Philosophy*, vol. 2, trans. E. B. Ashton (Chicago: University of Chicago Press, 1970), 45–46, 93–94.

32. See Ludwig Wittgenstein, *Tractatus Logico-Philosophicus*, 5.61.

33. See Novak, *Jewish Social Ethics*, 163–66.

34. See Immanuel Kant, *Critique of Practical Reason*, 1.2.2.4.

35. See B. Sanhedrin 5b regarding II Chron. 19:6.

36. See David Novak, *Covenantal Rights* (Princeton, N.J.: Princeton University Press, 2000), 13–14.

37. See Brian Tierney, *The Idea of Natural Rights* (Atlanta: Scholars Press, 1997), 33–34, 214–15.

38. See Kant, *Groundwork of the Metaphysic of Morals*, 114–21.

39. See B. Yoma 67b regarding Lev. 18:4.

40. See Maimonides, MT: Sanhedrin, 24.1.

41. Maimonides, MT: Berakhot, 11.2.

42. See B. Pesahim 106a.

43. *Kesef Mishneh*, on Maimonides, MT: Berakhot, 11.2.

44. See Maimonides, MT: Melakhim, 8.11.

45. No doubt for that very reason, there were rabbis who did require blessings to be recited before the performance of commandments with human objects. See T. Berakhot 6.9 and Saul Lieberman, *Tosefta Kifshuta: Zeraim* (New York: Jewish Theological Seminary of America, 1955), 112.

46. See B. Taanit 21a.

47. Indeed, claimants are obligated to make their claims publicly (proclaim), lest it be thought that they were compliant in the crimes being committed against them. See Nahmanides, *Commentary on the Torah:* Deut. 22:22–24; see also B. Baba Kama 91b regarding Gen. 9:5.

48. See Novak, *Covenantal Rights*, 131–43.

49. See B. Shabbat 127a regarding Gen. 18:3.

50. This principle is used in the Talmud (B. Avodah Zarah 27a regarding Gen. 17:13, and parallels) to explain why, infrequently, the Torah seems to use too many words to make a point (based on the assumption that normally each word has one or more meanings rather than one meaning coming from two or more words; see, e.g., B. Sanhedrin 34a regarding Ps. 62:12 and Jer. 23:29; *cf.* Abraham Ibn Ezra, *Com-*

mentary on the Torah: Num. 23:7, ed. A. Weiser [Jerusalem: Mosad ha-Rav Kook, 1977]). Maimonides, following Ibn Ezra (see Maimonides, *Commentary on the Torah:* Exod. 13:17, 19:20, 20:1) among others, uses this principle to explain why the Torah often had to use anthropomorphisms in speaking of God (see Maimonides, *Guide of the Perplexed*, 1.26). I use this principle here, however, to explain why the Torah and the Jewish tradition usually teach ethics in a way that is already intelligible to any rational, morally earnest, human being.

51. Israel Lipschuetz, *Tiferet Yisrael*, on M. Baba Batra 10.8.

52. *Digest*, 1.1.10.1, quoted in Frier, *Casebook on the Roman Law of Delict*, v. See *Mekhilta de-Rabbi Ishmael:* Mishpatim, ed. H. S. Horovitz and I. A. Rabin (Jerusalem: Wahrmann, 1960), 266, regarding Deut. 25:3; Maimonides, *Sefer ha-Mitsvot*, neg. no. 300; MT: Hovel u-Maziq, 5.1.

53. M. Ohalot 7.6; B. Sanhedrin 72b; Y. Shabbat 14.4/14d.

54. M. Sanhedrin 4.5. For the correct reading of the Mishnah here, see Louis Ginzberg, *Legends of the Jews*, vol. 5 (Philadelphia: Jewish Publication Society of America, 1925), 67, n. 8.

55. Kant, *Groundwork of the Metaphysic of Morals*, 95–98.

56. See the statement of the Union of Orthodox Jewish Congregations of America (www.ou.org/publicstatements/2005/n//.htm), which uses almost the same logic as the United Synagogue of Conservative Judaism (http://uscj.org/stem cell-research_a6675.html) and the Union for Reform Judaism (http://urj.us/cgi-bin/resodisp.pl). See also the testimony of Rabbi Elliot Dorff (Conservative) and Rabbi Moses Tendler (Orthodox) before the National Bioethics Advisory Committee in June 2000 (www.bioethics.gov/stemcell3.pdf).

57. For a full discussion of current Jewish views on abortion, both religious and secular, see Daniel Schiff, *Abortion in Judaism* (Cambridge: Cambridge University Press, 2002), esp. 227–69.

58. See Elliot Dorff, *Matters of Life and Death* (Philadelphia: Jewish Publication Society, 1998), 129–33.

59. See Maimonides, MT: Rotseah, 1.9, based on B. Sanhedrin 72b and Y. Shabbat 14.4/14d. See also Novak, *Law and Theology in Judaism*, vol. 1, 114–24.

60. See B. Baba Metsia 62a regarding Lev. 25:36.

61. See M. Sanhedrin 8.7; B. Sanhedrin 73a regarding Lev. 19:16.

62. See B. Yevamot 12b regarding Ps. 116:6.

63. See B. Sanhedrin 57b regarding Gen. 9:6; ibid. 59a and Tos., s.v. "leeka."

64. See B. Baba Kama 46b.

65. This section is largely based on Novak, *Natural Law in Judaism*.
66. For a full study of this institution, see David Novak, *The Image of the Non-Jew in Judaism* (New York and Toronto: Edwin Mellen Press, 1983).
67. See Novak, *Jewish Social Ethics*, 22–36.
68. For one of the earliest uses of this term, which nonetheless conceptualizes much earlier scriptural and rabbinic norms, see Saadiah Gaon, *Book of Beliefs and Opinions*, trans. S. Rosenblatt (New Haven, Conn.: Yale University Press, 1948), 3.1.
69. This is the title of Heschel's greatest theological statement: *God in Search of Man* (New York: Farrar, Straus, and Cuddahy, 1955).
70. Note B. Berakhot 57b: "The [experience of] the Sabbath is one sixtieth of the world-to-come." For the universality of the final redemption, see, e.g., Isa. 56:7; Zeph. 3:9; T. Sanhedrin 13.2 and B. Sanhedrin 105a regarding Ps. 9:18; Maimonides, MT: Melakhim, 8.11.
71. This is somewhat akin to what Hegel, influenced (as he surely was) by Jewish eschatology (however mediated by Christian theology), meant when he saw the culmination of the history of the Spirit to be in the total coming together of what is concrete (*an sich*) and what is abstract (*für sich*). See *Phänomenologie des Geistes*, ed. J. Hoffmeister (Hamburg: Felix Meiner Verlag, 1952), 20–21, 549–56.
72. B. Sanhedrin 59a.
73. *Cf.* Joseph Albo, *The Book of First Principles*, 3.13–14.
74. See Kant, *Critique of Pure Reason*, B46–59.
75. See B. Sanhedrin 57b; Maimonides, MT: Melakhim, 9.14.
76. That commandment also includes special moral obligations to fellow members of the sinaitic covenant (*benei brit;* see M. Baba Kama 1.3), such as the prohibition of taking interest on a loan to a fellow covenant member and the prohibition of paying interest on a loan from a fellow covenant member (see M. Baba Metsia 5.11; B. Baba Metsia 75b) because he or she is "your brother" (Lev. 25:36) and because God is the "father" of this extended family. See Mal. 2:10 and Rashi's and Ibn Ezra's comments thereon; see also Novak, *Jewish Social Ethics*, 223–24.
77. Aharon Lichtenstein, "Does the Jewish Tradition Recognize an Ethic Independent of Halakha?" in *Modern Jewish Ethics*, ed. M. Fox (Columbus: Ohio State University Press, 1975), 65.
78. For the Noahide duty to rescue human life endangered by a murderer or a rapist, see Maimonides, MT: Melakhim, 9.4 and 14.
79. I translate *ha'adam*, literally "the man," as "humankind" because *ha'adam* includes both the male (*ish*) and female (*ishah*) genders. See

B. Eruvin 18a regarding Gen. 5:2; see also B. Yevamot 61a regarding Num. 19:14 and Tos., s.v. "v'ein" (the view of Rabbenu Tam).

80. Regarding the punishment fitting the crime, see Y. Berakhot 1.5/3c regarding Exod. 20:13 and Deut. 11:17. Regarding killing another human as an assault on God, see *Mekhilta de Rabbi Ishmael:* Yitro, ed. Horovitz and Rabin, 223, regarding Exod. 20:13; *Zohar:* Yitro, 2:90a.

81. See B. Sanhedrin 54a regarding Lev. 18:7.

82. To be sure, human embodied being does not depict a divine body (see Maimonides, MT: Yesodei ha-Torah, 1.8). Humans are created in the image of God (*be-tselem elohim*—Gen. 1:26; 5:1; 9:6), which means they reflect rather than depict their unique connection to God, which is unlike that of any other creature. This connection is like the rays of the sun: From the experience of these rays alone, one could not even imagine what the sun itself looks like (see B. Hullin 59b–60a). All one knows is that something greater than these rays is casting them. See B. Shabbat 50b regarding Prov. 16:4 and Rashi, s.v. "bi-shvil qonehu"; see also Novak, *Natural Law in Judaism*, 167–73.

83. See David Hume, *A Treatise of Human Nature*, 3.1.2.

84. B. Sanhedrin 56b regarding Gen. 9:6.

85. See *Mekhilta de-Rabbi Ishmael:* Yitro, ed. Horovitz and Rabin, 232.

86. Thus, the commandment to warn one's fellow human person not to commit a sin that this person is just about to commit (see B. Yevamot 65b re Prov. 9:7) is an act of *imitatio Dei*.

87. Thus, when scripture speaks of God "commanding" nonhuman nature (e.g., Ps. 33:9, 148:5–6; Job 38:10–11), it seems to be using a metaphor because nature appears to be functioning in an orderly, obedient, lawful manner. Accordingly, the attempt to derive divine commands from the lawlike behavior of nonhuman nature is an erroneous derivation of an *ought* from an *is*. But *cf.* B. Eruvin 100b.

88. For the difference between human free choice (*behirah hofsheet*) and divine creative will (*ratson*), see Maimonides, *Guide of the Perplexed*, 2.18 and 2.48.

89. See David Novak, *Halakhah in a Theological Dimension* (Chico, Calif.: Scholars Press, 1985), 96–101.

90. See Emmanuel Levinas, *Totality and Infinity*, trans. A. Lingis (Pittsburgh: Duquesne University Press, 1969), 96–101.

91. The one exception to the notion that only God or humans as the image of God can make just moral claims upon each other might be the law prohibiting cruelty to animals (*tsa'ar ba'alei hayyim;* see B. Shabbat 128b; B. Baba Metsia 32a–b regarding Deut. 22:4). One could say that this law gives normative expression to the just claim of

another sentient being: "Do not harm me!" (see B. Baba Metsia 85a regarding Ps. 145:16; Maimonides, *Guide of the Perplexed*, 3.26 and 3.48.) Nevertheless, the difference between our relations to animals and our relations to fellow humans is that we would not know what animals are claiming from us unless we first had experience of what humans claim from us. In other words, in essence we only know animal claims upon us by analogy; we know human claims, however, directly inasmuch as most of them are spoken to us. That is why some commentators have taken scriptural stories about animals making verbal claims on humans (e.g., Gen. 3:1–5; Num. 22:28) to be fables or dreams. See the view of Saadiah Gaon mentioned in Ibn Ezra, *Commentary on the Torah:* Gen. 3:1; Maimonides, *Guide of the Perplexed*, 2.42.

92. Hence, humans have to be commanded not to violate God's created natural order. See B. Sanhedrin 60a and Tos., s.v. "huqqim."

93. See Maimonides, *Commentary on the Mishnah:* Hullin 7.6 regarding B. Makkot 233b.

94. See *Mekhilta de-Rabbi Ishmael:* Mishpatim, ed. Horovitz-Rabin, 263, regarding Exod. 21:14; see also Meir Simhah of Dvinsk, *Meshekh Hokhmah:* Exod. 21:14.

95. B. Sanhedrin 57b. Note also B. Niddah 30b, where in one version of a case (*cf.* T. Niddah 4.17), Rabbi Ishmael rejects the halakhic value of results drawn from an experiment that involved an abortion (see *infra*, 81–82, n.110). One could say that Rabbi Ishmael's rejection of this evidence was a result of the immoral way this experiment was conducted as well as the immoral character of the persons who conducted it. (For the invalidity of evidence provided by persons of questionable moral character, see M. Sanhedrin 3.3; Maimonides, MT: Edut, 10.1-111.22, and esp. B. Gittin 28b; B. Niddah 45a; Y. Pesahim 8.6/36a regarding Ps. 144:8.)

96. For similar exegesis about a life within a life, see B. Hullin 72a regarding Num. 19:13.

97. For this type of retrospection, taking a scriptural verse to be alluding to rather than grounding a norm already known, see, e.g., B. Sanhedrin 22b regarding Ezek. 44:7.

98. See B. Yoma 85a.

99. MT: Melakhim, 8.11.

100. See Novak, *The Image of the Non-Jew in Judaism*, 288–94.

101. *Cf.* Spinoza, *Tractatus Theologico-Politicus*, chap. 5.

102. MT: Melakhim, 9.1.

103. See Rashi, *Commentary on the Torah:* Gen. 40:9.

104. B. Sanhedrin 58a.

105. For the greater gravity of an act of commission than that of the inaction of omission, see B. Yevamot 90a–b and Rashi, s.v. "shev v'al ta'aseh"; B. Sanhedrin 58b and Rashi, s.v. "qoom aseh."

106. See Moshe Tendler, "Rabbinic Comment: In Vitro Fertilization and Extrauterine Pregnancy," *Mount Sinai Journal of Medicine* 51 (1984): 8–9; Haim David Halevi, "Fetal Reduction" (Heb.), *Assia* 47–48 (1990): 15. *Cf.* J. David Bleich, "In Vitro Fertilization," *Tradition* 25 (1991): 97.

107. See Dorff, *Matters of Life and Death,* 66–97.

108. See, e.g., B. Sanhedrin 78a and Tos., s.v. "mar."

109. This might be the type of scriptural verse that the rabbis assumed to be speaking about what is normally the case, yet not confining the verse's prescription to these examples alone. See *Sifre:* Devarim, no. 255 re: Deut. 23:11; M. Baba Kama 5.7/B.; Baba Kama 54b, and Rashi, s.v. "be-hoveh."

110. The first case, at B. Hagigah 14b–15a, deals with a woman who was impregnated in a bathing pool (*ambati*) by sperm from the semen of a man who had ejaculated into the pool while bathing there just before the woman's entrance there. The only question the Talmud raises about this case is whether this woman, who was a virgin, retains her virginal status because she was impregnated without having engaged in an act of normal sexual intercourse. See Immanuel Jakobovits, *Jewish Medical Ethics: A Comparative and Historical Study of the Jewish Religious Attitude to Medicine and Its Practice,* new ed. (New York: Bloch Publishing Co., 1975), 246–48. To my knowledge, no commentator even suggests that a baby so unusually conceived may be killed. The second case, at B. Sanhedrin 65b, tells of the Babylonian sage Rava, who "created a man" whom he sent to Rav Zeira for examination. When this creature cannot answer Rav Zeira, he is told by Rav Zeira to die—which could mean that Rav Zeira actually killed him. Rav Zeira's reason is that this creature is a magical entity and did not really come from a human source. Nevertheless, the late-seventeenth-century halakhist Zvi Ashkenazi (*Sheelot u-Teshuvot Hakham Zvi,* no. 93) argues that if this creature demonstrated any human purpose (*to'elet*)—which seems to mean if it could demonstrate any line of recognizably human development—it should not be killed, regardless of its unusual origins. Following this logic, I would say that any entity, however and wherever it was conceived, that possesses its own unique human DNA also possesses the human right to life, unless it

forfeits that right by directly threatening another human life—which could only be the life of the mother carrying it within herself.

111. M. Ohalot 7.6.

112. B. Sanhedrin 72b, Rashi, s.v. "yatsa r'osho." See also B. Niddah 44b and Rashi, s.v. "nefashot" regarding Num. 19:18. *Cf.* Elijah Gaon of Vilna (Gra), *Commentary on the Latter Prophets:* Isa. 9:5 (Jerusalem: Feldheim, n.d.).

113. B. Sanhedrin 59a. See also B. Yevamot 22a.

114. See, e.g., B. Baba Kama 83a regarding Num. 10:36.

115. See David Novak, *Covenantal Rights* (Princeton, N.J.: Princeton University Press, 2000), 128–31.

116. As a child of eleven, I heard this story from my maternal grandmother, Leah Eller Wien (d. 1953). With tears in her eyes, my grandmother told me of the sadness of the whole family that this choice had to be made; she told me that this sadness was like that of the family over the death by scalding in 1895 of three-year-old Louis, my great-grandmother's fourth child, whom my grandmother still called after all those years "our little brother." The baby who had to be aborted also was a boy, which made the comparison to Louis more poignant, although I am sure the tragedy would have been just as painful if the baby had been a girl. All the children in my great-grandparents' house, boys or girls, present or departed, were loved.

117. See Plato, *Phaedo*, 64D–67C. *Cf.* B. Berakhot 10a; *Vayiqra Rabbah* 34.3 regarding Prov. 11:16

118. See Gen. 1:20–21, 24; 2:6; Lev. 11:46.

119. See B. Gittin 23b and parallels. The principle that "the fetus is its mother's limb" (*ubar yerekh immo*) is cited twelve times in the Babylonian Talmud. For the debate over the applicability of this principle, whether it involves human life or animal life, see B. Sanhedrin 80b and Tos., s.v. "ubar." Moreover, even if the fetus is only its "mother's limb," aborting it for any reason other than to save the mother's life would minimally constitute prohibited self-mutilation. See B. Baba Kama 91b; Hayyim Yair Bachrach, *Sheelot u-Teshuvot Havot Yair*, no. 163 regarding Deut. 4:15.

120. See Maimonides, MT: Mamrim, 2.4 for the analogous use of this norm.

121. *Cf.* the note of J. Theodor and C. Albeck in their edition of *Beresheet Rabbah* 34.10, p. 321. A difficult counterexample to the general prohibition of abortion appears in M. Arakhin 1.4, which states that execution of a pregnant woman for a capital crime is not to be postponed except when she is already in labor, just about to deliver

her baby. The Talmud (B. Arakhin 7a) states that this prohibition obtains because after the baby has begun to descend in the birth canal it is considered to be a "separate body" (*gufa aharina*). Nevertheless, one cannot infer from this most unusual case (because Jews were not practicing capital punishment at the time these texts were composed, this case is hypothetical only) any permission to kill a fetus that has not yet become "its own body." In fact, on the same page of the Talmud (ibid., 7a–b), there is a mandate to violate the Sabbath if doing so is necessary to save a fetus that is still in utero. Moreover, there is the talmudic principle not to generalize from the laws of judicial punishment to nonpunitive situations (see B. Sanhedrin 54a and parallels; *Encyclopedia Talmudit*, 1:321–24, s.v. "ein onshin min ha-din").

122. M. Niddah 5.3.

123. B. Niddah 44b.

124. A woman who has aborted her unborn child—like anyone else who aborted an unborn child, even accidentally—apparently is obliged to pay damages (the amount of which is to be determined by the court) to the father of this unborn child, whoever he is, provided he could prove his paternity. See M. Baba Kama 5.4; T. Baba Kama 9.20; Y. Baba Kama 5.5/5a; B. Baba Kama 49a regarding Exod. 22:23. See also *Shemot Rabbah* 30.6 regarding Ps. 99:8 and David Luria, *Hiddushei Radal* thereon regarding Job 33:16; Maimonides, MT: Isurei Biah, 10.12 regarding M. Niddah 3.4.

125. See B. Shabbat 129a and parallels.

126. B. Sanhedrin 59a. For the best attempt to synthesize the various talmudic rulings concerning abortion into one consistent general norm, see Ezekiel Landau, *Sheelot u-Teshuvot Noda Bi-Yehudah* (Jerusalem: n.p., 1960), vol. 2, Hoshen Mishpat, no. 59.

127. B. Sanhedrin 59a, Tos., s.v. "leeka."

128. B. Berakhot 62b regarding I Sam. 24:10; B. Sanhedrin 72a; see also ibid., 82a. Note *Digest*, 9.2.4pr: *nam adversus periculum naturalis ratio permittit se defendere*. Ibid., 9.2.45.4: *vim enim vi defendere omnes leges omniaque permittit*.

129. Cf. B. Pesahim 25b.

130. M. Eruvin 7.11. Unlike monetary benefit, which an unwitting beneficiary could reject, denying *post factum* that it really is to his or her benefit (see B. Baba Batra 138a and Rashbam, s.v. "k'an" regarding Prov. 15:27; Yom Tov ben Abraham Ishbili, *Hiddushei ha-Ritva* [Warsaw: n.p., 1902]: Kiddushin 23a), one may not waive his or her right to be rescued from death any more than one may waive his or her

right to be spared any bodily harm (see M. Baba Kama 8.7; see also B. Kiddushin 19b and Rashi, s.v. "bi-dvar she-be-mamon").

131. B. Sanhedrin 72b; Y. Shabbat 14.4/14d. See Maimonides, MT: Rotseah, 1.6.

132. B. Baba Metsia 62a; see also *Sifra:* Behar, 109c, regarding Lev. 25:36. See Novak, *Covenantal Rights,* 125–31.

133. For talmudic discussion of whether something is a matter of exegesis (*qra*) or a matter of reasoning (*sevara*) and, if a matter of reasoning, why the exegesis is needed, see B. Shevuot 22b and Tos., s.v. "iba'it eima qra."

134. B. Sanhedrin 9b and parallels.

135. See ibid.; Tos., s.v. "v'ein."

136. For another example of the proximity principle as it applies to rescue from harm, see B. Baba Metsia 71a regarding Exod. 22:24.

137. B. Pesahim 25b.

138. M. Ohalot 7.6. For further discussion of what constitutes "most" of the fetus extra utero, see T. Yevamot 9.4.

139. B. Sanhedrin 72b.

140. MT: Rotseah, 1.9. Regarding "in the hands of Heaven" (*bi-yedei shamayim*) as a synonym for natural causality as distinct from artificial, human production (*bi-yedei adam*), see, e.g., M. Negaim 11.3 and Maimonides, *Commentary on the Mishnah* thereon.

141. See B. Sanhedrin 73a.

142. Y. Shabbat 14.4/14d. The parallel text at Y. Sanhedrin 8.9/26c asks what we are to do when the pursuer (*rodef*) becomes the pursued (*nirdaf*) and vice-versa.

143. B. Yevamot 90a. *Cf.* Maimonides, MT: Melakhim, 9.14.

144. See Eliezer Waldenberg, *Tsits Eliezer,* 2nd ed. (Jerusalem: n.p., 1985), vol. 7, no. 48, chap. 1, 190–91.

145. See B. Berakhot 60a.

146. B. Sotah 2a. See B. Nazir 51b and Tos., s.v. "keivan"; B. Menahot 99b and *Bemidbar Rabbah* 5.5 regarding Deut. 25:3 and 9.1; *Beresheet Rabbah* 32.5 regarding Gen. 7:4; *Tanhuma:* Naso 6, ed. M. Buber (Jerusalem: n.p., 1964), 15a regarding Num. 5:2; *Vayiqra Rabbah* 23.12 regarding Job 10:3; M. Keritot 1.5 and Maimonides, *Commentary on the Mishnah* thereon.

147. See Novak, *Law and Theology in Judaism,* vol. 1, 9–14.

148. See Zvi Hirsch Chajes, *Darkhei Horaah,* sec. 2, *Kol Kitvei Maharats Chajes* 1 (Jerusalem: Divrei Hakhamim, 1958), 251–52. *Cf.* Menahem ha-Meiri, *Bet ha-Behirah:* Baba Batra 130b, ed. B. Menat (Jerusalem: n.p., 1971), 382 regarding Y. Peah 2.4/17a.

149. B. Sanhedrin 91b regarding Job 10:12 and Meir Abulafia, *Yad Ramah* thereon regarding Gen. 21:1 (*cf.* B. Niddah 16b regarding Job 3:2). Some modern Jewish scholars dogmatically dismiss the text at B. Sanhedrin 91b as having no halakhic value. See D. M. Feldman, *Birth Control in Jewish Law* (New York: New York University Press, 1968), 274–75 and n. 44 thereon; Jakobovits, *Jewish Medical Ethics*, 376, n. 138. Nevertheless, although a nonlegal text cannot establish a norm, it can help determine a legal fact. See B. Baba Kama 2b and parallels. Note that the forty-day criterion, which is based on an *aggadah*, is invoked for halakhic purposes by some scholars who no doubt would dismiss the *aggadah* about human life beginning at the time of conception. Why is one aggadic definition halakhically valuable and the other not?

150. B. Yevamot 69b. See Maimonides, MT: Terumot, 8.3.

151. In the *Bavli*, the term *b'alma* designates a physical substance that has no definite function in a particular context, even though it might have a definite function in another context. See, e.g., B. Zevahim 42b and Tos., s.v. "ki"; B. Hullin 97b–98a and Alfasi, *Digest:* Hullin, 35a. Earlier, the Mishnah (M. Zevahim 8.9) refers to something "as if it were water" (*k'ilu hen mayyim*) in the same way. This text might be the origin of the term *maya b'alma*.

152. In a discussion in the *Bavli* (B. Niddah 24b regarding M. Niddah 3.3) that is pertinent to the question of whether fetal material is "mere water," the first assumption is that a woman who delivers a watery substance in lieu of a recognizable human baby has delivered "nothing" (*u-mayyim lo klum hi*)—that is, what she has delivered has no recognizable human properties. Yet in subsequent discussion (ibid., 25a), opinions are cited that hold that if this watery substance is cloudy (*akhur*), it might have some human properties (*tsurat adam*—see M. Niddah 3.1), thus requiring further purification rites by the woman who delivered it (see Y. Niddah 3.3/50d). Maimonides, however, rejects this opinion (MT: Isurei Biah, 10.10 and Vidal of Tolosa, *Maggid Mishneh* thereon).

153. See Aristotle, *History of Animals*, 7.3/583b1-20; see also Jakobovits, *Jewish Medical Ethics*, 174–75; Feldman, *Birth Control in Jewish Law*, 266, n. 82.

154. See Peter Singer, *Unsanctifying Human Life*, ed. H. Kuhse (Oxford: Blackwell, 2002), 184–87.

155. See B. Sanhedrin 46b and Y. Nazir 7.1/55d regarding Deut. 21:23.

156. This commandment includes restoring one's lost health, even if, in the case of innovative therapies such as those that use stem cells, that

"restoration" is projective rather than retrojective. See B. Sanhedrin 73a regarding Deut. 22:2; Maimonides, *Commentary on the Mishnah: Nedarim* 4.4.

157. For another use of the term *maya b'alma* by Rashi, in a case that does not involve human life, see B. Hullin 64b and Rashi, s.v. "mutarot."
158. M. Bekhorot 8.1/B. Bekhorot 47b, Rashi, s.v. "le-yom arba'im."
159. Ibid.
160. M. Keritot 1.5/B. Keritot 7b, Rashi. s.v. "ha-mapelet"; B. Bekhorot 21b, Rashi, s.v. "arba'im yom." See also M. Niddah 3.7/B. Niddah 30a, Rashi, s.v. "einah hoshevet le-vlad"; M. Ohalot 18.7 and Maimonides, *Commentary on the Mishnah* thereon. *Cf.* B. Niddah 57a and Rashi, s.v. "la beq'ei be-yetsirah" thereon.
161. Along these lines, note that a child who dies before reaching the age of thirty days after birth is not to be the object of formal mourning rites (*avelut*). With regard to formal mourning, this child is considered a stillborn child (*nefel*)—or, one might say, like "mere water." See T. Shabbat 15.7; B. Shabbat 135b regarding Num. 18:16; B. Niddah 44b; Y. Tevamot 11.7/12b; *Bemidbar Rabbah* 4.3 regarding Num. 3:40; *Shulhan Arukh: Yoreh Deah*, 374.8; Y. Y. Greenwald, *Kol Bo al Avelut* (New York: Feldheim, 1965), 199–200. Yet no one could or should infer from this legal fact any permission to kill such a nonviolable child, even when that fact is known *ab initio*. See M. Niddah 5.3; B. Niddah 44b regarding Lev. 24:17.
162. M. Hullin 10.4; B. Hullin 134a and Rashi, s.v. "halah" thereon; Y. Halah 3.4/59b; M. Tahorot 4.12; B. Baba Kama 46a regarding Exod. 24:14.
163. See B. Baba Batra 127a; Maimonides, MT: Nahalot, 2.6.
164. See Maimonides, MT: Bikkurim, 11.19.
165. See B. Niddah 25a and Rashi, s.v. "le-humra."
166. See Lev. 12:8 and 6:22; M. Zevahim 6.4.
167. Like most rabbinical criteria of differentiation (see, e.g., M. Hullin 8.3), the forty-day criterion seems to be empirical rather than scientific—a direct inference from ordinary experience rather than a precise measurement that has been experimentally validated. For the empirical criteria for differentiating the stages of pregnancy, see B. Yevamot 37a and Rashi, s.v. "li-shlish yamim regarding Gen. 38:4; ibid., 42a–b.
168. According to the Talmud (B. Niddah 72b), the shortest time between two menstrual periods is 11 days. If the average woman menstruates every 28 days, a miscarriage around the fortieth day after the first missed period could be misconstrued as the onset of a period or the onset of nonmenstrual vaginal bleeding (*zavah*).

169. See B. Baba Kama 118a.
170. See B. M. Carlson, *Patten's Foundations of Embryology* (New York: Mc-Graw Hill, 1996), 3.
171. B. Yoma 85b.
172. Ibid.
173. Moses Nahmanides, *Torat ha'Adam:* Inyan ha-Sakkanah, *Kitvei Ramban*, vol. 2, ed. C. B. Chavel (Jerusalem: Mosad ha-Rav Kook, 1963), 28–29, based on *Halakhot Gedolot:* Yom ha-Kippurim, vol. 1, ed. E. Hildesheimer (Jerusalem: Mekitse Nirdamim, 1971), 319–20 and its reading of B. Shabbat 151a and B. Yoma 82a. See also B. Niddah 44a–b, Tos., s.v. "ihu" (second opinion). For the opinion that this applies only when the fetus's life is intertwined with that of its mother (which, of course, is not the case with an embryo that is extrauterine), see Rabbenu Asher, *Rosh:* Yoma, 8.13 regarding Rashi at B. Yoma 82a, s.v. "ubrah" (M. Yoma 8.5); Nissim Gerondi (Ran), Commentary on *Alfasi:* Yoma, Vilna ed., 3b; Joseph Karo, *Bet Yosef* on *Tur:* Orah Hayyim, sec. 517. See also Saul Lieberman, *Tosefta Kifshuta:* Moed (New York: Jewish Theological Seminary of America, 1962), 246. Nevertheless, one should not infer from proscribed rescue in a certain case permission to actively kill what may not be rescued in that case. On this overall point, see B. Avodah Zarah 26a–b and Tos., s.v. "ve-l'o moridin."
174. Only in certain matters involving rabbinic legislation is one permitted to violate the law when great loss is at stake. See B. Ketubot 60a; *Shulhan Arukh:* Orah Hayyim, 336.9.
175. See B. Sanhedrin 79a and parallels; ibid., 78a; Maimonides, MT: Rotseah, 2.7–8. For the principle that what is exempt from humanly administered punishment (*patur*) is still forbidden (*asur*), see B. Shabbat 3a; Y. Horayot 1.1/45b and Mosheh Margolis, *Pnei Mosheh*, s.v. "ve-hen she-horu muttar" thereon; B. Niddah 44a–b and Zvi Hirsch Chajes, *Hagahot ve-Hiddushim* thereon. In other words, one is not to derive a norm from a fact—even a legal fact. Cf. Hume, *A Treatise of Human Nature*, 3.1.1.
176. See T. Shabbat 15.5; B. Shabbat 135a; B. Yevamot 80a–b and Rashi, s.v. "mipnei ha-sakkanah" thereon; *Shulhan Arukh:* Even ha'Ezer, 156.4 and note of Moses Isserles (Rema) thereon. See also M. Makhshirin 6.7 and Maimonides, *Commentary on the Mishnah* thereon; Maimonides, MT: Melakhim, 9.4.
177. See, e.g., M. Baba Kama 9.1 and B. Baba Kama 96b; see also M. Baba Kama 1.1 and B. Baba Kama 6a. Cf. M. Hullin 3.1 and B. Hullin 54a.
178. See Kant, *Groundwork of the Metaphysic of Morals*, 95–96.

179. See Novak, *Jewish Social Ethics*, 22–44.
180. For the recognition that ritual matters have their own legal criteria, see B. Berakhot 19b and parallels; B. Ketubot 46b and parallels.
181. See M. Hullin 3.1; T. Hullin 3.19; Maimonides, MT: Maakhalot Asurot, 4.8–9.
182. MT; Shehitah, 10.12–13. In *Kesef Mishneh* thereon, Joseph Karo locates Maimonides' talmudic source as B. Hullin 54a. However, Maimonides also adds his own explanation by quoting Deut. 17:11: "according to the instruction [*torah*] by which they [the rabbis] instruct you." The knowledgeable reader will remember the end of that verse: "You shall not depart from what they will tell you either to the right or to the left," and its best known rabbinic interpretation, "even if it appears to you that what they say is left is really right and what they say to you is right is really left, listen to them" (*Sifre: Devarim*, no. 154, ed. L. Finkelstein [New York: Jewish Theological Seminary of American, 1969], 207; see the note of my late revered teacher, Louis Finkelstein, thereon). Note also that the opposite interpretation of this verse appears at Y. Horayot 1.1/45d—namely, that one should heed the rabbinic tradition only when what the rabbis say is right really is right and what they say is left really is left. In other words, one should accept only what the rabbis present as rationally convincing. Perhaps we could resolve the conflict between these two interpretations by applying the former to ritual matters (as Maimonides did here) and the latter to interhuman matters.
183. MT: Shehitah, 10.12–13.
184. B. Hullin 10a. See T. Hullin 3.19; M. Terumot 8.6; Y. Terumot 8.3/46a; Maimonides, MT: Rotseah, 11.5 (see also Maimonides, MT: Deot, 4.1).
185. See B. Sanhedrin 78a.
186. Maimonides, MT: Rotseah, 2.8. For an example of where current scientific opinion is sought in an area of Jewish law pertaining to interhuman relations, see T. Niddah 4.3–4; B. Niddah 22b.
187. See Maimonides, *Commentary on the Mishnah:* Berakhot 5.3, following Saadiah Gaon, *Book of Beliefs and Opinions*, 3.1. Cf. *Commentary on the Mishnah:* Avot, intro. (*Shemonah Peraqim*), chap. 6; Maimonides, *Guide of the Perplexed*, 3.26.
188. See Abravanel, *Commentary on the Torah:* Shoftim, q. 5 regarding Deut. 17:1.
189. See Novak, *Natural Law in Judaism*, 99–105.
190. See e.g., B. Sanhedrin 90a–b.
191. See Novak, *Law and Theology in Judaism*, vol. 2, 106–8.

192. See Deut. 21:23; B. Sanhedrin 46b; Y. Nazir 7.1/55d; T. Eruvin 2.6; B. Eruvin 17a.

193. See B. Yoma 85a regarding Gen. 7:2; see also B. Taanit 2b regarding Gen. 2:7.

194. See, e.g., Gen. 3:19; Ps. 30:10; Eccl. 12:7.

195. See Baruch Brody, *Abortion and the Sanctity of Human Life* (Cambridge, Mass.: MIT Press, 1975), 107–12.

196. See B. Shabbat 129a and parallels; see also B. Yoma 85a.

197. See M. Avot 4.1 regarding I Sam. 2:30.

198. See n. 176.

199. *Sheelot u-Teshuvot Havot Yair*, no. 31. Along these lines, see *Sefer Hasidim*, Bologna ed., no. 1101.

200. See B. Sukkah 29b–30a regarding Mal. 1:13; B. Sanhedrin 6b regarding Ps. 10:3; Y. Hallah 1.5/58a (opinion of R. Yose); B. Shabbat 6a and Tos., s.v. "ve-khi"; see also *Septuagint* and *Targum Jonathan ben Uzziel* on Deut. 16:20.

201. See Maureen Condic, "Stem Cells and Babies," *First Things*, no. 155 (2005), 12–13.

202. M. Avot 2.16.

2

A JEWISH ARGUMENT FOR
SOCIALIZED MEDICINE

UNIVERSAL HEALTH CARE: CANADA AND
THE UNITED STATES

My concern with the question of socialized medicine, or universal health care, and a Jewish approach to it has been greatly heightened by my experience in Canada during the past ten years. I now hold citizenship in Canada as well as the U.S. citizenship conferred upon me by my birth in the United States. I proudly retain my U.S. citizenship because of what the United States has done for me and my family, going back several generations. I have not ceased to be an American, but as a Canadian I have a new basis for comparison of morally significant phenomena in my two countries.

As most readers know, Canada provides health care for all of its citizens and residents. Equally well known is that the United States does not provide universal health care. Approximately 40 million Americans are without any regular health care; these people must depend on the arbitrary charity of public and private institutions. That sad fact came home to me almost twenty years ago, when I had to take my wife to a hospital emergency room in New York City. There I saw the large number of poor people who had to use that emergency room as their primary health care facility—after the staff there could take time away from the paying patients. Many of their more serious health problems had to wait for treatment until my wife's less serious problem was treated—because she had health insurance and they did not. Either they never had any health insurance, or they had had it and lost it because it came with a job they had lost.

Despite all the problems Canadian health care services entail—such as having to wait almost a year for elective surgery, as I once did—I firmly believe that health care delivery in Canada is fundamentally just, and health care delivery in the United States is fundamentally unjust. As an American and a Canadian, the question I must address is why this belief is rationally justified. More important, however, as a Jew I must base this belief on the authoritative sources of the living Jewish tradition.

MORAL AND THEOLOGICAL PROBLEMS WITH THE PRACTICE OF MEDICINE

I begin by looking at a shocking rabbinic text that has embarrassed many Jews, especially because of the long Jewish involvement in medicine. The Mishnah states that Rabbi Judah said in the name of Abba Gurya, a man of Sidon, "The best of the physicians belongs in hell [*tov she-ba-rof'im le-gehinnom*]."[1] In his Talmud commentary, Rashi, the great eleventh-century French commentator, gives four reasons for this seemingly harsh judgment.[2] First, physicians are not apprehensive about disease and let sick people eat food that is only fit for healthy people. Second, physicians do not pray (literally, "break their hearts") to God. Third, physicians sometimes kill humans. Fourth, physicians have the power to heal poor persons yet often refuse to do so. Each of these reasons for a harsh indictment of ancient medicine could be applied to modern medicine as well.

PREVENTIVE MEDICINE

With regard to the first reason, Rashi is dealing with what one might consider preventive medicine. In ancient times, this practice was a much greater factor in medicine than it has been in modern times. Although Rashi was a medieval thinker, he was much closer to the ancient world than to the modern world, so he could identify with the situation of medicine in the ancient world that was assumed in the Mishnah more easily than we can identify with it.[3] In the ancient world, physicians probably focused as much (and perhaps more) on prescribing healthy living to their patients as on treating the bad effects of their patients' often unhealthy lives.[4] Today, except for the annual physical examination that most of us who are more than fifty years old get from our private physicians—or that insurance companies occasionally require us to undergo—most of us deal with physicians on a crisis basis. Rashi reminds us that physicians ought to be our teachers even before they are our rescuers. If preventive medicine was wanting in his day, how much more so is it in our day—when U.S. physicians, especially, are required by those who employ many of them to see more and more patients in less and less time.

RELIGIOUS MEDICINE

Rashi's second reason for the condemnation of physicians brings up a delicate problem, especially in a multicultural, secular society such as ours. Can we expect our physicians to pray? Of course, if one regards the practice of medicine as entirely mundane—no different, in essence, from having one's car repaired—then the relationship of the physician to God is unimportant. Yet few of us regard our bodies, which physicians treat, as commodities like our cars. We *are* our bodies, so we cannot truthfully treat them like mere things. To say I own my body is to say that I created or acquired my body, which is untrue. My body is not *mine;* it is *me.* It is personal and sacred; as such, it may not be violated or treated as any kind of commodity. Moreover, I cannot destroy my body without destroying myself. I am not related to my body as if it were something detachable from myself, like anything I have made or acquired. Therefore, either my body/myself has been purposely made by someone greater than myself and all those like me, or my body/myself is only an accident. If I regard my becoming what I am to be as an accident for which no one is responsible, however, how can I act purposefully and responsibly in such an absurd universe in which my own being is equally absurd? Certainly my own projects, my own self-created purposes, are not powerful enough to overcome the basic absurdity of the universe of which I am but a tiny part. Therefore, how the physician regards his or her own body/self is of great importance to how he or she considers my body/self. Our bodies and the bodies of all others have enough sanctity to dispel the notion that we are mere things, but not enough self-sufficiency to embrace the notion that we are gods. Because we did not make or acquire our bodies, they are not things. Because we did not make or acquire ourselves, we are not gods.

Because few of us regard our bodies as mere commodities, few of us would regard physicians, to whom we allow the most intimate access to our bodies next to that of our mates, to be mere mechanics. A physician comes closest to God in our experience of bodily dependence in the world. That relationship, of course, opens a physician to the temptation of thinking that he or she really is God. In fact, a large part of the current appeal of the field of biomedical ethics relates to our fear that physicians, because of the vast new power that comes from the expansion of medical technology, have been "playing God" in an unlimited way that is unbecoming for any mortal creature. We want physicians to be answerable to standards that are not of their own making—that is, not made by them for their own self-interest. That also explains the staggering cost of medical malpractice suits in the United States. Many observers believe that such suits are the only real check ordinary citizens have on what otherwise would be medical omnipotence. Perhaps the Jewish tradition had the "God-complex" temptation of physicians in mind when it occasionally made some negative remarks about medical practice.[5]

The irony is that the expansion of medical technology has made physicians much less likely to think of themselves as mechanics. Ironically, in our so-called secular age we use the term "miracle" more often than our supposedly more religious ancestors. How many times have we heard the term "medical miracle" used in ordinary discourse and the media? Hence, the issue is not secular versus religious medicine. When medical treatment is a serious matter of life and death, better questions are these: Whose God? Whose God is the physician's? Whose God is the patient's?

Many years ago, when I was a young rabbi, I visited a woman in a hospital on the day she was to have a life-threatening operation. I asked her how she felt, and she told me, "I have absolute faith in my doctor." She asked me if what she said was right, so I told her, "Save your absolute faith for God, trust your doctor, and hope he is doing God's work." She was a religious person, so she did not argue with me on that point. Not having met her physician, however, I cannot say whether I could have said something similar to him: "Have faith in God, don't betray your patient's trust, and hope you are doing God's work."

Nevertheless, most of us would not want to be treated by a physician who thinks he or she is God because that clearly is not true, and any physician who thinks he or she is God is not likely to have the patient as his or her prime concern. Such concern with the patient would interfere with the physician's own self-worship. People who lie to themselves are in a bad position to be truthful with others, which is to recognize these others for what they truly are. Instead, such a physician will be much more concerned with his or her "God-like" reputation.[6] The best physician for the patient is one whose concern for the patient is greater than his or her power over the patient. Patients and their physicians should regard themselves as participants in a process that no human creature has been able to initiate or will be able to conclude. No human creature has the Creator's unique power to create life or to create life beyond death. That understanding best prepares patients to expect only partial care and even more partial cure from their physicians, and it prepares physicians to expect only partial success in their treatment of their patients. After all, life itself can be regarded as a terminal disease. Even if a miracle—meaning something beyond our normal expectations—does occur, the physician is its conduit, not its creator. Hence, at a minimum we would want a physician who does not think he or she is God and therefore does not expect worship from us. In other words, medicine should avoid idolatry— which for Judaism is the sin of all sins.[7] Moreover, the patient and the physician are part of the same process, and the preeminence of the physician over the patient is a difference of degree, not a difference in kind. They are both members of the same species, not only biologically but morally and spiritually as well.[8]

Maximally, from a Jewish perspective, the opposite side of the negation of medical idolatry should be that both the physician and the patient have a positive relationship with God—what Judaism would call a covenant. In a secular or even multicultural society, however, such a covenant is not something a patient can require of his or her physician or a physician can require of his or her patient. Conversely, rejection of idolatry is indeed something any human can ask of any other human. It is rationally demonstrable. In other words, one can say that from the very meaning of the name God—even if one is not sure there really is a God—it is obvious that human persons are not God. A positive relationship with God can come only from the acceptance of God's revelation to a particular community in history. In truth, one cannot argue someone else into faith the way one can (at least potentially) argue someone else out of idolatry. Only the God who reveals Himself in a historical event can elicit faith from people who have experienced that event directly or people who, having heard about this event, feel as if they were there as well and respond accordingly.[9] Even the coercion of a good argument will not work. Therefore, even in a secular context, where we cannot assume our physician will be of our faith or any faith, we can still be wary of the physician whose faith is in himself or herself and expects similar devotion from his or her patients.

CARELESS MEDICINE

Rashi's third reason for the condemnation, "The best of the physicians belongs in hell" is because physicians can and do kill. Of course, Rashi could be referring to medical carelessness: the type of malpractice we all dread, when the physician has not taken the proper precautions in treating the perilous situations in which patients often find themselves.[10] Such situations are the stuff of malpractice suits, which now so often elide the difference between human fallibility and human culpability. Nevertheless, taking Rashi's comment as not only insightful but prescient, we are reminded of the situation today in which some physicians have insisted that they have a duty to enable patients to end their lives in voluntary death, just as they have always had a duty to enable patients to continue their lives voluntarily. This transformation of physicians from angels of life into angels of death, which turns them into executioners as well as practitioners, contravenes all of our traditions about medicine.[11]

For most of us, medicine should always be maximally about saving human life, minimally about comforting human life, but never about deliberate termination of human life.[12] (Physicians who perform non-life-saving abortions are in this category too.[13] I would even place in this category physicians who administer lethal injections for the state in cases of capital punishment.) This new situation, however, is a corollary of the divinity some of us have invested in our technologically advanced physicians. Like all false gods, the "creator" is actually the creature. As such, the real creator, which is now human projection, can demand of its divinized creature, which is modern medicine, that it deliver what its creator wants—even if what it wants is a request for self-immolation. Idolatry is involved here as well because one would only turn one's body over to the life-and-death power of a person if one considered that person a god. The other alternative—the physician as mechanic—does not explain the fascination of a Dr. Jack Kevorkian.

COMMERCIAL MEDICINE

Rashi's fourth reason for the condemnation of physicians brings us directly into our topic, which deals with how society authorizes and funds medical treatment for its citizens and residents. I have analyzed Rashi's first three reasons for the Mishnah's condemnation of physicians because I believe all four reasons hang together in a logical sequence. That is, ignoring preventive medicine can lead to the notion of medicine as essentially miraculous intervention in a crisis, and this attitude can lead a physician to regarding his or her death-bringing powers as on a par with his or her life-bringing powers—that is, the physician may exercise medical power in the most powerful way, for life or for death. Finally, that perspective can lead one to regard the practice of medicine as being the type of entrepreneurship practiced by the pagan gods, which meant soliciting more and more opulent offerings from their worshipers in return for favors granted.[14] (The ordinary mechanic, who promises only ordinary services, usually gets more ordinary reimbursement from his or her customers.)

MEDICINE AS A SACRED PROFESSION

Rashi's condemnation of medicine as commerce seems to presuppose that there is a prohibition against physicians selling their services. Thus, they have no right to withhold their services from patients who cannot pay. Where, however, is this prohibition actually stated? A principle of Jewish law holds that one may not be condemned for committing a sin unless that sin has been already prohibited.[15] Furthermore, if there is such a prohibition, is there also an imperative for one to become a physician? Who, then, may not sell his or her services on a quid pro quo basis?

There is a specific scriptural prescription to save a human life, even if doing so requires intervention on the part of the rescuer: "You shall not stand idly by your neighbor's blood" (Leviticus 19:16)—which means that you shall intervene by all means possible to save someone else's life if it is in danger.[16] This prescription is considered a positive commandment of the Torah. Like all commandments of the Torah pertaining to interhuman relations, there is a right and a correlative duty. There is a claim to which there is a required response.[17] The right or claim is that of the person in mortal danger. This right is that person's claim on whoever has the power and opportunity to rescue him or her from mortal danger to do so unconditionally. The duty or response rests with the person who has the power and opportunity to rescue the person who is mortally threatened. The Torah recognizes the right to be rescued from harm and thus commands rescue as a duty to be performed by whoever is capable of doing so. The question is: May one claim reimbursement for his or her performance of the duty of rescue?

There is a principle in the Talmud that answers this question. "The commandments [*mitsvot*] are not given for monetary benefit."[18] In other words, no one is to be paid for performing his or her duty, whether that duty is owed to God or to another human being. Hence, if the practice of medicine is a performance of the duty of rescue, physicians—and, in fact, everyone we call health care professionals—may not receive compensation for their services.

We might ask, however: Is one expected to lose money in the performance of his or her divinely mandated duty? Would physicians not be losing money by performing their duty without compensation? Would the performance of this duty without charge not keep them from otherwise earning a living? Some rabbis teach that one's sole reward for performing a commandment is to be found in the world to come, not in this world.[19] Yet should someone else benefit from my regularly performing a commandment on their behalf in this world, while I am penalized for it by being prevented from making a living because of it? In the case of acts not specifically mandated by the Torah, I can accept payment for services rendered without any such theological impediment.

At the most extreme level, no human being has the right to ask another human being to die for him or for her.[20] At most, one human being has the right to die for another human being if he or she so chooses.[21] To make such a choice is commendable, but not to make that choice carries no penalty. Accordingly, not only does no human being have the right to be rescued at the expense of the rescuer's life, no human being has the right to even deprive another human being of the rescuer's property that was used in rescuing himself or herself from death. For example, if saving my life requires the destruction of some of your property, I have the right to destroy your property. You certainly do not have the right to withhold your property from me if it is needed to save my life.[22] Nevertheless, you also have the right to compensation from me for your monetary loss.[23] Another example: Although there is a duty to give charity to poor persons, the rabbis decreed that this charity should not amount to more than 20 percent of one's annual income—because one's generosity should not impoverish oneself or one's family.[24]

If that is the case, why can't the physician say to the patient, "As I am benefiting you with my services, you should benefit me by contributing to my support by paying my fee"? How is such an agreement any different from the grocer who rescues me from starvation by supplying me with food, for which nobody suggests I should not pay him or her (if I have the money to do so)? Nevertheless, Jewish law follows the opinion of the great thirteenth-century Spanish-Jewish theologian-jurist Nahmanides (himself, like many of the medieval rabbis, a physician), who stated, "As for the matter of payment for medical services [*sekhar refu'ah*], my opinion is that it is permitted to accept payment for the time and effort expended [*sekhar betalah ve-tirha*] but not payment for the actual medical prescription [*sekhar ha-limud*] since that involves the possible loss of life, and the Torah says 'you shall return to him [what he has lost—Deuteronomy 22:2].' As for the performance of any commandment [*mitsvah*], it is to be for free [*be-hinam*]."25

Yet how can one distinguish between the effort expended in the practice of medicine and the actual practice itself, which is a prescription of one kind or another? Furthermore, the notion of payment for the time one expends is my own loose translation of the Hebrew *sekhar betalah*, which literally means "payment for doing nothing." In other words, we are supposed to be paying the physician for not doing something other than conducting his or her medical practice. That position assumes, however, that we know what a physician would be doing if he or she were not a physician, as well as what he or she would be willing to accept for being idle by not doing it.26 Considering the amount of time and effort required to become a physician, however, the actual calculation of what this other profession might pay him or her, let alone what he or she would accept for not engaging in it, seems to be highly imaginative precisely because these alternatives do not exist. Therefore, to make the *professional* distinction between a grocer and a physician a real difference, we need to regard the practice of medicine as by no means an ordinary job—even an ordinary job that benefits other people.

In the carefully worded text quoted above, Nahmanides states that he is expressing his own opinion. In rabbinic parlance, that means that he has no explicit source for what he believes the law to be. Nonetheless, he cannot simply create a law *de novo*. As a rabbi he has no *prima facie* authority.27 Therefore, his opinion must be an inference he has made from an authoritative source in either the Bible or the Talmud (of which the Mishnah forms the basic text). Nahmanides' source is a statement in the Mishnah about judges who take money from litigants who stand before them seeking justice.28 The Mishnah rules that their judgments are null and void because, as one of the major commentators points out, this situation is considered to be akin to the violation of the biblical commandment, "you shall not take a bribe" (Deuteronomy 16:19).29 In the ensuing discussion in the Talmud, the reason for this ruling is traced back to a statement of Moses: "See I have taught you [statutes and ordinances] which the Lord my God commanded me" (Deuteronomy 4:5). From this the Talmud infers, "Just as I taught you for free, so you should teach for free."[30] Of course, Moses' authoritative teaching is what Jews call *hora'ah*.[31] As the verse itself states, it is authoritative because it comes from God. Moses is able to teach for free because of what God gave him for free, not as a reward for his righteousness but as a message for the people to whom he is privileged to be God's messenger. In the Jewish tradition, Moses is the archetypal rabbi; he is called *Mosheh Rabbenu*, "Moses our Teacher," whose rabbinical authority is primarily juridical. (In traditional Jewish communities, the primary—indeed, essential—function of the rabbi is still that of judge, even though rabbis have always performed "clerical" duties as well.)

MEDICINE AS A CALLING

What do rabbis and physicians have in common to the exclusion of other socially useful professions? Each profession is meant to be a calling (*vocatio*)—that is, they are not mandated by ordinary commandments. Thus, in the case of saving human lives, the commandment "You shall not stand idly by the blood of your neighbor" (Leviticus 19:16) applies to anyone who happens to be in a situation in which he or she can save somebody else's life. Where, however, is one commanded to prepare for and devote himself or herself to the *profession* of saving lives—a profession that clearly will take all of one's time and energy? Based on the definition of the practice of medicine as a uniquely commanded activity, Nahmanides writes, "Any physician who knows this science and art [of medicine] is obligated [*hayyav hu*] to heal, and if he prevents himself from doing so, he has shed human blood."[32]

Although everyone is commanded to save a human life whenever and wherever possible, in dedicating oneself to medicine as one's profession one should regard himself or herself as if he or she had been *individually* called by God. Why? Because the profession of healing, the ongoing activity of being a physician, is an individual case of imitation of God (*imitatio Dei*).[33] In the Torah God says about himself, "I am the Lord your physician" (Exodus 15:26). That is why, it seems, the Talmud refers to the individual practice of medicine as being a "dispensation [*reshut*] that is granted [*nitnah*] to the physician to heal."³⁴ Who gives this dispensation? God—the author of the law of the Torah, who also is the arch-physician. It is a dispensation because without it one might think that the human practice of medicine is usurping a uniquely divine role in the world.³⁵

That reasoning also might explain why the practice of medicine is not called a commandment (*mitsvah*). That is, it can be experienced only by someone who believes himself or herself to be individually addressed by this imperative. Hence, we apply to it the word *reshut*, which often means an option one can choose or not choose with legal impunity.³⁶ Unlike ordinary commandments, there is no way anyone else can tell whether somebody has been so "commanded." Whether one feels called to be a professional participant in the divine process of healing is too intimate a matter to be the subject of a general commandment. It is almost idiosyncratic.

Here we can further develop the comparison of a physician to a judge. There is a general commandment to practice justice—"Justice, justice you shall pursue" (Deuteronomy 16:18)—which the Talmud interprets to mean seeking out the best possible judges.³⁷ Nevertheless, there is no general commandment for one to be a judge. That too is an individual case of the imitation of God because in the Torah God also is designated as "the judge [*ha-shofet*] of all the earth" (Genesis 18:25). In other words, just as a judge must feel individually called to heal the body politic to be adequate to the sanctity of the human community, a physician has to feel individually called to heal the human body to be adequate to its sanctity. Moreover, absent the notion that in the act of true judgment the judge becomes, in the words of the Talmud, "a partner [*shutaf*] in the work of cosmic creation," the execution of justice becomes more and more mundane, more and more a matter of mere social utility.³⁸

Furthermore, the comparison of a physician to a judge is helpful in justifying universal health care—which means, among other things, that physicians do not work for fees paid to them directly by their patients, or even by private insurers of their patients, for services rendered. In the case of judges, if they were to be paid by the persons who appear before them seeking justice, the judges would be in violation of the prohibition against taking bribes. Therefore, the Talmud answers that the judges in Jerusalem, who dealt with civil disputes involving Temple property, were paid out of Temple funds.[39] Later jurists argued that this payment of judges by the community, which made them civil servants, was the arrangement in the vast majority of Jewish communities everywhere. As the great twelfth-century French theologian-jurist Rabbenu Jacob Tam pointed out, judges are not paid by litigants, and the community is obligated to pay them because they have no other source of income.[40] An approximate contemporary of Tam's, Rabbi Judah the Barcelonan, mentions a special fund set designated by the community for that purpose.[41]

Interestingly enough, on the same page of the Talmud where this distinction between private and public payment of judges is being worked out, there is a reference to the fact that physicians do take fees from their patients, and the text associates this practice with the sin of taking bribes.[42] This reference probably means that the community had much more control over the allocation of justice than it did over the allocation of medical services. Jewish physicians probably were competing with non-Jewish physicians in a larger social context in which there was no such thing as physicians as communal employees. Nonetheless, following the comparison of medical practice with judicial practice, if a community does have the power to institute universal health care—which means making it a public service rather than a private option—it behooves the community to do so for its members.

Like judges, physicians are supposed to be licensed by the community.[43] Licensing, or communal authorization, is another meaning of the Hebrew word *reshut*—which when used for theological purposes refers to the divine dispensation for physicians to participate in what is taken to be the superhuman process of healing. I am examining its legal meaning, however. If the community believes it has the right to license persons who administer either justice or healing, does it have the right to refrain from so doing? I think not. Therefore, this authorization of persons who are doing God's work more directly than others appears to be a social duty. Could we not infer that this social duty also should include paying the salaries of health care professionals as a regular retainer?[44] In our day, we might ask: Given that society funds all kinds of medical research because this research eventually will benefit all of its citizens, does society not have a prior duty to fund medical treatment for all of its citizens—which will benefit them much more immediately? Only a society that had no money for medical research, no National Institutes of Health, could say in good faith that it had no such duty or that it could not fulfill such a duty.

Following the comparison with the administration of justice, could we not say that just as the administration of justice—protection of citizens from possible harm by other persons and rectification of real harm from other persons—is society's unique duty, shouldn't the delivery of health care—protection of citizens from possible harm from impersonal sources and rectification of real harm from impersonal sources—also be society's unique duty? Where there is injustice, some citizens are harmed by criminals, which might not be the case if there were better social controls.[45] Where there is a lack of universal health care, some citizens are harmed by disease, which might not be the case if there were better social treatment of disease. Although this analogy may seem farfetched, recall that the greatest medieval theologian-jurist-physician, Maimonides, compared a fetus threatening the life of its mother in utero to a criminal threatening the life of his or her victim.[46] Putting aside the question of whether the fetus is what we would call a person in Jewish law, certainly in utero the fetus is functioning impersonally.[47] Unlike the literal pursuer (*rodef*), the "pursuing" fetus has neither intelligence nor will. Yet we can still compare the personal and the impersonal, protection from injustice and protection from disease. (In other words, the life-threatening fetus is considered to be like a diseased organ of the mother's body that, if need be, must be amputated to save her life.)

NONSECTARIAN MEDICINE

The last question to address is the following: What does all of this information and reflection from the Jewish tradition have to do with the health care situation in the United States today? Why should anyone in a multicultural, secular society be bound by anything the Jewish tradition says? To answer this question positively, one must make two essential distinctions: the distinction between commandments that could be addressed only to Jews and commandments that could be addressed to any human being and the distinction between governance by one's own law and guidance from somebody else's.

The Jewish philosophical tradition makes a distinction between "rational commandments" (*mitsvot sikhliyot*) and "revealed commandments" (*mitsvot shim'iyot*).[48] Some theologians have noted that virtually all of the commandments that pertain to interhuman relations are in the category of rational commandments—that is, commandments that are readily acceptable to ordinary human reasoning and do not require that one affirm any singular revelation in history by becoming part of the community that has accepted that historical revelation.[49] For example, Maimonides rules that the benediction (*berakhah*) Jews recite before most commandments stating that God is the One "who has sanctified us by His commandments by commanding us to" do such and such is not said before the performance of any commandment that is done for the direct sake of another human being.[50] Maimonides did not think these commandments have a human source, rather than the divine source of all the commandments. Instead, he seems to have thought that the more direct source of these commandments is what human reason can directly discover about the legitimate claims of one human being upon another—although God, of course, is the ultimate source of these commandments.[51] Hence, some of what the Jewish ethical tradition puts forth might indeed make a moral claim on rational persons created in the image of God—that is, humans whose lives are sacred and whose reason is meant to determine how that sanctity is to be affirmed and enhanced in interhuman relations.

Even if one does not regard the Jewish ethical tradition as making any moral claims upon oneself, however, it still might inform one's moral decision making, even if only by analogy. In other words, the Jewish ethical tradition may offer some moral guidance, even if in principle it does not claim obedience from anyone who is not part of that tradition and in fact cannot morally claim obedience from anyone who does not want to be a part of that tradition.[52] Indeed, an ancient Jewish legend indicates that the Torah was given in the wilderness, in a place that belonged to no one (*hefqer*), because God wanted the nations of the world to be able to partake of it.[53]

The Torah was given twice, however: once at Mount Sinai shortly after the Israelites left Egypt and again on the Plains of Moab just before the Israelites were to enter the Promised Land. At this second giving of the Torah, the people were commanded to write it on stones for all to see (Deuteronomy 27:8). In this version of the legend of the Torah as being more than just for Israel, the nations of the world sent notaries to copy the Torah for themselves.[54] How much of the Torah was written for them to copy, however? One rabbi said all of it. Conversely, another rabbi said, "They only wrote what the nations would want."[55] This second rabbi gives an example regarding how to conduct oneself in war to avoid bloodshed if possible. According to the first rabbi, by copying all of the Torah the nations were now to be judged for their noncompliance with its governance. But if the Torah that was written for them was only the part of the Torah that would appeal to their rational will, it was only a source of guidance for them. As such, they were, in the words of the Talmud, "those who did even when not actually commanded to do so."[56]

Nevertheless, many people would consider general benevolence, including reverence for human life, morally obligatory for all humans.[57] Jewish tradition (especially its legal component), with its greater specificity, provides non-Jews with guidance regarding how to fulfill what they are more generally obliged to do.

Even if only in terms of guidance or counsel, the Jewish ethical tradition has much to offer people who want health care to be based on something more morally elevated than medicine as the practice of individual autonomy or the heteronomy of collective ownership of human persons. Judaism seems to have a third alternative, which is neither the capitalist notion of medicine nor the socialist one. Neither of these alternatives is sufficient to ground the respect for the sanctity of the human person as the image of God that is so rationally appealing. That is why the Jewish ethical tradition, which is based on this respect for the sanctity of human personhood, both individual and communal, is so attractive—if only for its insights rather than its authority; if only for its guidance rather than its governance.[58]

NOTES

The following abbreviations for classical Jewish sources are used throughout these notes:

B.   *Babylonian Talmud (Bavli)*

M.   *Mishnah*

MT   *Mishneh Torah* (Maimonides)

T.   *Tosefta*

Tos. *Tosafot*

Y.   *Palestinian Talmud (Yerushalmi)*

Unless otherwise noted, all translations are by the author.

1. M. Kiddushin 4.14.
2. B. Kiddushin 82a, s.v. "tov she-ba-rof'im."
3. See Rashi, *Commentary on the Torah:* Exod. 15:26.
4. In Aristotelian terms, the first type of medical practice is a form of distributive justice—namely, who deserves or needs what. The second type of medical treatment is a form of corrective justice, restoring what originally belonged to someone and had been taken away. See *Nicomachean Ethics*, 5.2-4/1130b–1132a19. I invoke this idea to prepare the reader for the analogies between the practice of medicine and the practice of justice I discuss subsequently in this chapter.
5. See, e.g., II Chron. 16:12; M. Pesahim 4.9. *Cf. Sirachides* 38:1–14.
6. For a modern critique of this whole mindset, see Robert Mendelsohn, *Confessions of a Medical Heretic* (Chicago: Contemporary Books, 1979), 123–40.
7. See B. Kiddushin 40a regarding Jer. 6:19.
8. See Benjamin Freedman, *Duty and Healing* (New York and London: Routledge, 1999), 152–86.
9. See B. Shevuot 39a and *Tanhuma:* Nitsavim, no. 8, ed. S. Buber (Jerusalem: n.p., 1964), 25b, regarding Deut. 29:13.
10. For notions of medical malpractice in rabbinic sources, see T. Gittin 3.8; T. Baba Kama 9.11. As we shall soon see, physicians are compared to judges. For questions pertaining to judicial malpractice, see B. Sanhedrin 5a, 33a.

11. See *infra*, 111–27.
12. See B. Shabbat 151b; see also David Novak, *Law and Theology in Judaism*, vol. 2 (New York: KTAV, 1976), 98–106.
13. See B. Sanhedrin 57b regarding Gen. 9:6; ibid. 59a and Tos., s.v. "leeka;" David Novak, *Law and Theology in Judaism*, vol. 1 (New York: KTAV, 1974), 114–24.
14. See Plato, *Euthyphro*, 14D–15A.
15. B. Sanhedrin 54a–b.
16. See B. Sanhedrin 73a; see also Maimonides, MT: Rotseah, 1.5 regarding M. Sanhedrin 4.5.
17. See David Novak, *Covenantal Rights* (Princeton, N.J.: Princeton University Press, 2000), 3–12.
18. B. Rosh Hashanah 28a.
19. B. Kiddushin 39b regarding Deut. 5:16 and 22:7. *Cf.* Tos., s.v. "matnitin" thereon.
20. B. Baba Metsia 62a regarding Lev. 25:36; the view of Rabbi Akivah is to be followed in any dispute he had with a colleague (see B. Eruvin 46b and parallels).
21. See Y. Terumot 8.4/46b; see also David Novak, *Jewish Social Ethics* (New York: Oxford University Press, 1992), 111–14.
22. B. Sanhedrin 73a.
23. B. Sanhedrin 74a; see also M. Baba Kama 10.4. *Cf.* Maimonides, MT: Hovel u-Maziq, 8.14.
24. B. Ketubot 50a; see also T. Arakhin 4.24–26. Even when performing commandments that are duties owed to God, where one is required to spend his or her money for the objects involved in these acts, one is not required to impoverish oneself because of them. See M. Negaim 12.5; M. Keritot 1.7; T. Niddah 9.17; see also B. Shabbat 118a; Maimonides, MT: Shabbat, 30.7.
25. *Torat ha'Adam:* Inyan ha-Sakkanah, in *Kitvei Ramban* 2, ed. C. B. Chavel (Jerusalem: Mosad ha-Rav Kook, 1963), 44. The talmudic source for the analogy of returning lost property and restoring life is at B. Sanhedrin 73a.
26. M. Baba Metsia 2.9.
27. See B. Menahot 29b.
28. M. Bekhorot 4.6.
29. B. Bekhorot 29a and Tos., s.v. "mah" regarding B. Ketubot 105a.
30. B. Bekhorot 29a.
31. See Y. Berakhot 4.5/8c regarding II Chron. 3:1.
32. *Torat ha'Adam*, 42.

33. Even the attendance to the need of the sick (*biqqur holim*) that is required of ordinary nonprofessionals is considered to be *imitatio Dei*. See B. Sotah 14a regarding Gen. 18:1. Cf. Maimonides, MT: Evel, 14.1 regarding Lev. 19:18. Nevertheless, this *imitatio Dei* is not an individual option.

34. B. Baba Kama 85a regarding Exod. 21:19. The Hebrew term *reshut* has several meanings in rabbinic literature. For its meaning as a dispensation from what would ordinarily be forbidden, see T. Maasrot 2.14. Sometimes, such a dispensation is called a benefit or an entitlement (*zekhut*). See B. Baba Metsia 89b.

35. See Nahmanides, *Commentary on the Torah*: Lev. 26:11; *Torat ha'Adam*, 42, regarding B. Berakhot 60a; see also David Novak, *The Theology of Nahmanides Systematically Presented* (Atlanta: Scholars Press, 1992), 83–87.

36. See, e.g., M. Shevuot 3.6.

37. B. Sanhedrin 32b.

38. For the notion of human partnership with God the creator, see B. Shabbat 119b regarding Gen. 2:1.

39. B. Ketubot 105a. See M. Sheqalim 4.1.

40. B. Ketubot 105a and Tos., s.v. "gozrei gezerot;" see also B. Bekhorot 29a and Tos., s.v. "mah."

41. *Tur*: Hoshen Mishpat, 9.

42. B. Ketubot 105a regarding Deut. 16:19.

43. T. Baba Kama 9.11.

44. For the implication that a community is obliged to provide certain social services, including having a physician in residence, see B. Sanhedrin 17b. For the notion that the community has the right to determine where a physician in its midst may and may not practice medicine, see B. Baba Batra 21a; *Tur*: Hoshen Mishpat, 156; and Joseph Karo, *Bet Yosef* thereon.

45. See Y. Sotah 9.6/23d.

46. MT: Rotseah, 1.9 regarding B. Sanhedrin 72b.

47. M. Ohalot 7.6. Cf. M. Niddah 5.3.

48. See Saadiah Gaon, *Book of Beliefs and Opinions*, 3.3.

49. See M. Baba Batra 10.8 and Israel Lifschuetz, *Tiferet Yisrael* thereon, n. 84.

50. MT: Berakhot, 11.2, and Joseph Karo, *Kesef Mishneh* thereon.

51. See B. Yoma 67b regarding Lev. 18:4; see also David Novak, *Natural Law in Judaism* (Cambridge: Cambridge University Press, 1998), 89–91; see also *supra*, 31–35.

52. See B. Shabbat 88a.
53. *Mekhilta de-Rabbi Ishmael:* Yitro, ed. H. S. Horovitz and Rabin (Jerusalem: Wahrmann, 1960), 205, regarding Exod. 19:1.
54. To.: Sotah 8.6.
55. Quoted from Saul Lieberman, *Tosefta Kifshuta:* Nashim (New York: Jewish Theological Seminary of America, 1973), 700.
56. B. Kiddushin 31a and parallels.
57. See, e.g., Maimonides, *Commentary on the Mishnah:* Peah 1.1 regarding B. Shabbat 31a.
58. Thus, if one wants to be under the authority of the Jewish tradition, one should convert to Judaism (see Maimonides, MT: Melakhim, 10.9); that decision is not a moral necessity, however. Indeed, that is why one can choose not to convert to Judaism with moral impunity (see B. Ketubot 11a). That also is why, according to Maimonides (MT: Melkahim, 8.10), Jews are to enforce moral law among non-Jews over whom they have political control. Yet Jews are forbidden to force Judaism on any non-Jews as a necessary moral option, which is not the case with fellow Jews (see Maimonides, MT: Gerushin, 2.20; see also B. Ketubot 86a–b).

3

PHYSICIAN-ASSISTED SUICIDE

THEOLOGY, PHILOSOPHY, AND POLITICS

Following the procedure of the preceding chapters, I deal with the question of physician-assisted suicide in three contexts: theological, philosophical, and political. In fact, the separation of these three contexts of the normative discussion of this question can be more precisely maintained here than in the preceding chapters because the theological discussion of this question need not be largely constructed anew, on the heels of the philosophical arguments, so to speak. The sources that are pertinent to the overall question of suicide and the question of agency that is so central to the question of appointing a physician to help a person commit suicide are very evident and extensive in the Jewish tradition. As such, for the most part they need representation rather than construction *de novo*. Conversely, the theological sources that are pertinent to a question such as universal health care and certainly to a question such as stem-cell research are much less evident and extensive in the Jewish tradition. In contrast to the two preceding chapters, we can make the transition from theology to philosophy and then to politics more easily in this chapter because we can more easily begin with theology.

As a theologian, I begin with theology because my primary existential and intellectual commitment lies there. I can begin there with greater ease because I need not first confront the normative question at hand in a philosophical context, as was the case with stem-cell research (because that question initially arose in a philosophical context). Similarly, I need not first confront the normative question at hand in a political context, as was the case with universal health care (because that question initially arose in a political context). In dealing with the normative questions of the two preceding chapters, I had to continually work backward into theology, either from the philosophical discussion or from the political discussion. Therefore, in those chapters, the logical sequence of the discussion often had to be different from its rhetorical sequence. In this chapter, however, the logical sequence of the discussion and the rhetorical sequence run together for the most part.

WHO IS GUILTY IN PHYSICIAN-ASSISTED SUICIDE?

The moral judgment about the act of physician-assisted suicide largely depends on how the act of suicide itself is judged. Physician-assisted suicide presupposes suicide, but suicide itself does not necessarily entail a physician's assistance. In fact, most suicides are truly reflexive acts (the *sui* in *suicide*); they are committed without any outside assistance.

So why would anyone want someone else's assistance, whether that person is a physician or not, for an act that the person almost always can commit quite easily himself or herself? I return to this question later in this chapter when I examine what the motivation might be for seeking assistance in committing suicide. That motivation might be different from the motivation in seeking assistance in committing homicide—the act to which suicide most often is compared if not actually subsumed. One's intention in committing suicide and seeking assistance in doing so is different, however—phenomenologically, if not legally—from one's homicidal intention and one's intention in seeking assistance from others in committing murder.

To begin, however, I look at the legal connection in Judaism between suicide and a physician's assistance in committing it. I then locate precisely the derivation of the prohibition of suicide—because suicide is not explicitly prohibited in scripture. Homicide, on the other hand, is explicitly prohibited in the Decalogue: "Thou shalt not murder" (Exodus 20:13; Deuteronomy 5:17). Suicide and homicide obviously are closely related acts, yet there are some significant differences between them.[1]

Both homicide and suicide are prohibited in the Jewish tradition. Legally, they differ only in terms of the punishment they entail as sins or crimes. Of course, if every suicide is judged after the fact to have been psychotic behavior—which most if not all Jewish jurists now take for granted—there is no punishment for what is regarded as behavior that was induced by forces that truly overwhelmed the self-destructive person himself or herself.[2] Whether the suicide was really beyond the control of the now-deceased person who killed himself or herself, however, is left to the judgment of God in and for the world-to-come—as is the case with all human acts committed in this world.[3] Legally, the greatest difference between suicide and homicide is that whereas we now judge all suicides to have been accidental, we still judge homicides to have been premeditated (*zadon*), careless (*shegagah*), or accidental (*ones*).[4] To be sure, nowhere today do Jewish religious courts have the power to adjudicate cases of homicide in the sense of being able to actually punish murderers and manslaughterers.[5] Nonetheless, we can make a moral distinction (that is, one that is not humanly punishable) between an act of suicide and an act of homicide. We still judge these two acts differently, in moral terms if not in terms of legal consequences.

The fact that suicide is prohibited in the Jewish tradition, even if it is never humanly punishable, is important. Secular systems of law have gone much further, however. Thus, in secular discussions of physician-assisted suicide, proponents and opponents can no longer assume that suicide is a crime (as it once was in English common law, for example). Therefore, proponents of physician-assisted suicide can argue that there is no rationale for prohibiting suicide and penalizing any physician who assists a patient in committing suicide, inasmuch as the physician is not an accomplice in any crime.[6] Conversely, opponents of physician-assisted suicide in the political context of a secular society, with secular law as their only public point of reference on the issue, cannot argue against it directly. They can argue against it only for two less direct reasons.

First, the tradition of medical ethics, going back to Hippocrates, prohibits physicians from killing their patients, whether directly or as accomplices. Second, physician-assisted suicide inevitably involves situations in which physicians are not simply agents carrying out the directives of their autonomous patients; these patients are more likely to be complying with the autonomous directives of their physicians to cooperate with the physicians in their own demise.[7] I return to this point later in dealing with the question of whose agent the physician really is. Is the physician representing the patient who employed him or her or the state that has authorized him or her to practice medicine in its domain and carry out its public policies there?

Emphasizing either reason for prohibiting physician-assisted suicide—from medical tradition or from fear of abuse of patient autonomy—opponents of physician-assisted suicide can only criticize either what seems to be an ethical indiscretion on the part of the assisting physician or the possibly inadequate judgment of the patient. Proponents of physician-assisted suicide, conversely, are proposing no direct violation of any law, although the practice must be regarded as a radical innovation nonetheless.

With regard to Jewish law, there are no posthumous penalties (in this world, at least) for a successful suicide; nevertheless, no one who is contemplating suicide can justify this act to himself or herself by assuming that God has permitted his or her suicide, let alone mandated it. (The only exception would be martyrdom, and the Jewish tradition has tried to make as sharp a difference as possible between martyrdom and suicide.)[8] Compliance with a non-crime, therefore, is not a problem Jewish theologians need to face when they are explaining to their own community why physician-assisted suicide is morally wrong. Even though all suicides are now regarded, after the fact, as having been psychotic behavior, they are not considered permitted *ab initio* to anyone who is capable of making an intelligent moral choice and who, as such, is not psychotic by definition.[9]

For the Jewish tradition, the issue of whether the physician is acting on his or her own behalf or on behalf of the patient requesting assistance in committing suicide is irrelevant. Whether the act is instigated by a patient requesting assistance in ending a life he or she has no right to end or by a society that authorizes or even permits (which often amounts to unofficial authorization, in the form of approval or suggestion) a physician to end a patient's life, with or without the patient's subsequent consent, there is no difference from the Jewish perspective. Society has no right to kill an innocent person, even if its officials judge that such a death is good for the whole society.[10] That conclusion would obtain even in the case of comatose patients, when a physician kills a patient (either directly by "pulling the plug" or less directly by stopping feeding and hydration) by acting on what the physician or someone closest to the comatose patient thinks is what the patient would want if he or she were able to express a desire to die.[11] The sin (even if it escapes human punishment) is still that of homicide when it is directly committed by a physician—or anyone else, for that matter.

Thus, secular societies made a mistake when they decriminalized suicide, even though committing suicide should entail no penalties (such as public disgrace of the corpse of the suicide *post factum*) because the person suffering such penalties would not suffer the penalties; his or her family would.[12] (Of course, some persons, especially young persons, commit suicide precisely because of the emotional suffering—in the form of feelings of inner guilt and outward disgrace—their suicide will cause their family members, who they often think deserve to suffer because of how they abandoned the person to his or her own self-destruction.) Nevertheless, decriminalizing suicide was a political mistake (in the sense of being imprudent) because it pulled the rug out from under any attempt to criminalize assisted suicide as compliance with the commission of a crime. Where there is no crime, there can be no compliance with a crime; instead, we are left with a wrong that is less than compliance with a crime and often now entails little more than decreasing social stigma in most secular societies.

Even though observant Jews might live their lives governed by Jewish law, almost all of them live in secular societies and cannot help but be influenced by the prevailing secular mores there.[13] That reality seems to be a fact of social psychology. Moreover, changed secular attitudes toward suicides have had a great influence on secular systems of law, which do impinge on the lives of even the most religious persons inasmuch as such persons are members of secular societies and are governed by such systems of law in all civil and criminal matters. The decriminalization of suicide per se is the result of a mistaken notion of autonomy that has had great force in the social psychology and legal systems of secular societies today. I argue against this notion not only from a theological perspective but also from a philosophical perspective. (I discuss this point later when I consider the question philosophically.) How deeply one can argue against this notion politically, however—considering its already considerable effects in our secular societies—is very much a matter that calls for prudential judgment. (I discuss this point later when I consider the question politically.)

Neither society nor any individual is ever authorized to kill an innocent person, even when that innocent person commits the sin of requesting his or her own death.[14] The sin of requesting one's own death from another human being is not itself a capital crime for which one deserves to be killed by society, however; indeed, such a request does not seem to entail any humanly administered punishment at all.[15] Hence, the person who requests suicide is an innocent victim of the crime he or she is requesting be committed against him or her, even when that person thinks that being killed is for his or her own benefit or the benefit of others—or even when this person thinks he or she deserves to die. No one is authorized to instigate his or her own death at the hands of another, even if that other is society (except when the society is required by law to execute certain criminals). An individual person is authorized to kill another person only in a clear case of self-defense, as I discuss in chapter one of this volume.[16] I do not address the question of whether that justification also authorizes society to kill certain dangerous criminals or take vengeance on certain criminals; that would take me too far afield from the question at hand.

What we now call physician-assisted suicide involves one of five possible scenarios, all of which can be considered, at least *prima facie*, as being authorized by patients exercising autonomy over their own lives and deaths. These five scenarios are as follows:

- At the behest of the patient, or at the behest of someone who claims to know what the wishes of a comatose patient would be, a physician himself or herself causes the death of the patient—for example, by injecting the patient with a lethal dose of a drug.

- A physician orders someone under his or her authority, such as a nurse, to kill the patient similarly.

- A physician prescribes suicide for his or her patient, such as by telling the patient, "As your physician, I have determined that ending your life now is in your best interest and that of society, and this is how you can best do it."

- A physician provides a patient with the means for his or her own death, such as giving the patient poison or a lethal instrument that the patient can use to kill himself or herself.

- A physician indirectly advises a patient about how to kill himself or herself, such as telling the patient, "Remember, when you take the pills I have prescribed for you, an overdose will be fatal."

THE PHYSICIAN KILLS THE PATIENT

In this first scenario, the physician has committed homicide. This conclusion is evident in a much-discussed text in the Talmud: "It is taught that one who says to his agent [*le-shluho*]: 'Go and kill this person [*ha-nefesh*],' he is liable [*hayyav*], but his agent is not liable [*patur*]. Shammai the Elder said in the name of Haggai the prophet that his agent is liable as [scripture] says: 'You killed him with the sword of the Ammonites' (II Samuel 12:9)."[17]

The Talmud's discussion of this ancient tradition assumes that the first opinion (itself presented anonymously) is the view of the other rabbis; hence, "in the event of a dispute between one and many, the law is according to the many [*halakhah ke-rabbim*]."[18] Thus, Shammai the Elder is outvoted by his peers. (The Talmud's presentation of this dispute does not entertain the question of whether the peers of Haggai the prophet agreed or disagreed with him.)[19] Moreover, the discussion explicitly assumes that the principle "there is no agency for sin" (*ein sheliah li-dvar aveirah*) is indisputable; in fact, the Talmud cites the foregoing dispute to show that although this principle was debatable at one time, it is now beyond dispute and is taken to be a unanimous opinion.[20] The one who committed the act is primarily guilty, even when he or she is told to do so by someone else. In the case of physician-assisted suicide, the instigator is the patient who says to the physician, "Go kill this person," even though "this person" is the patient himself or herself. Therefore, the physician is guilty for having followed the illegitimate order of the patient. One does not have the legal power to delegate authority that one does not have to anyone else.[21] For all intents and purposes, the "agent" initiated the act himself or herself.[22]

One might infer from the foregoing text that the other rabbis do not ascribe any moral fault to the first party who instigates the murder of a third party by a second party. (In this case, the first party and the third party would be identical—namely, the patient who authorizes the physician to kill him or her.) Nevertheless, the Talmud is uncomfortable with this absolute dichotomy between the view of the rabbis and that of Shammai the Elder. It therefore narrows the difference by assuming that the rabbis do not consider the instigator of the act to be entirely innocent. The instigator is considered to be "slightly guilty" (*dina zuta*).[23] The great medieval commentator Rashi explains this explanation to mean that the instigator is "like an indirect cause" (*ke-gorem*) and thus deserves less punishment (presumably by God, in the world to come) than the actual perpetuator of the act.[24] Primary guilt (*dina rabba*) still belongs to the person who actually committed the act with his or her own body. Apparently, he or she is primarily guilty even if his or her crime was instigated at the request of the victim of the act.

THE PHYSICIAN ORDERS THE PATIENT TO BE KILLED

The second scenario, in which a physician orders someone under his or her authority to kill a patient (albeit with the prior authorization of the patient), appears to be the opposite of the first scenario. That is, whereas the acting physician is guilty of homicide in the first scenario, in the second scenario the physician's aide is guilty of homicide, having followed illegitimate orders—for which the aide is primarily responsible. Nevertheless, the late-fifteenth-century Jewish statesman and theologian Don Isaac Abravanel offers a striking reinterpretation of the scriptural prooftext brought by Shammai the Elder in the name of Haggai the prophet.[25] That prooftext comes from the rebuke of King David by Nathan the prophet for having ordered the death of Uriah the Hittite—the husband of his paramour, Bathsheba (later David's wife), whom in her husband's absence the king had impregnated. The king ordered his faithful servant, his general Joab, to place Uriah (who was one of Joab's soldiers) by himself into a battle situation against the Ammonites (who at the time were warring with Israel), where the foes would surely kill Uriah.[26]

Abravanel (based, no doubt, on his real political experience of the way royal power operates and the effect it has on the people over whom it has power) distinguishes between an ordinary order to kill someone and an order from a king to do so.[27] When an ordinary person "deputizes" someone, as it were, to kill somebody else in his or her behalf, that agent certainly has the power to resist such an order, which usually is more of a request. (This situation is akin to hiring a hit man to kill somebody; the hired killer can easily refuse to comply with this request.) The situation is decidedly different, however, when such an order comes from a king—who has the power of life and death over his all his subjects and certainly over all those who closely work with him on a regular basis.[28] (This situation would be akin to a mafia boss ordering one of his "soldiers" to kill a rival or another disloyal soldier.) In this case the agent has much less power to resist the king's orders, regardless of how unjust they might be, because the agent is terrified of the king and so terrorized by any of the king's orders that disobeying them would be virtually impossible for the agent. Questioning the orders of one's commander-in-chief, let alone refusing to obey them, simply is not part of such an agent's experience. (Moreover, Joab was so loyal to the king that he even killed David's rebellious son, Absalom, whom the king himself ordered to be spared; Joab was convinced that he knew what was in the king's best interest better than the king himself.)[29] Today we might remember that Nazi leaders were sentenced to death in the Nuremburg trials of 1946–47 for being responsible for the deaths of millions of innocent people, even though most of them pleaded innocent (*unschuldig*), claiming that they themselves had not actually killed anybody with their own hands.

In this way, Abravanel considerably narrows the dispute between Shammai the Elder and the other rabbis. That is, Shammai's view obtains when we have an unusual case such as that of David, Joab, and Uriah; the rabbis' view obtains when we have a more typical case involving a request from one ordinary person to another. Following Abravanel's lead, we might narrow the gap between Shammai's view and that of the other rabbis even further and make it more applicable to the issue of physician-assisted suicide. We might say that in any situation in which official orders—as opposed to an unofficial suggestion—are given, the official issuing the orders is almost as guilty as the underling who carries out these orders. There appears to be a closer connection between the sin of the physician who prescribes suicide to his or her patient and the sin of the patient who actually follows this prescription, often out of a sense of deference to medical authority rather than agreement with medical wisdom.

When the physician orders a nurse (or even an orderly) to kill a patient, the official orders come from the physician, even if they were originally instigated at the request of the patient. The nurse was doing what she or he did not because of the patient's request but because of the doctor's orders. Although in good conscience the nurse should have resisted the order (as have brave nurses who refuse to participate in unwarranted abortions), the doctor who ordered this killing is almost as guilty as the person who actually administered the lethal dose. Applying Abravanel's distinction (although Abravanel makes this distinction in an exegetical rather than a strictly legal context) to the case of a physician who orders an aide to kill a patient, we could say that the physician is doing much more than requesting an agent for sin. We could say that the physician is using that aide to kill the patient in the same way King David used the sword of the Ammonites—with Joab's compliance—to make Uriah's death a virtual certainty. Like Joab, this aide is unlikely to disobey the doctor's orders. Thus, in both the first and second scenarios, the physician is guilty of homicide—the difference in the physician's guilt being a matter of degree rather than kind.

Surely Uriah did not request his own death, however. Therefore, he is very different from the suicidal patient who requests a physician's assistance in killing himself or herself. In other words, the patient is more like King David, and the physician and the nurse are more like Joab.

In this context we confront the growing acceptance in secular societies of autonomy over oneself as a right to be enforced in law. That is, society increasingly assumes that I have a right to do with my own body whatever I choose to do with it, as long as I am not harming someone else.[30] My body is my possession, to do with as I choose. Moreover, because my body is my own possession, I am entitled to authorize someone else, as my agent, to do with my body or to my body what I have ordered that agent to do with it or to it. In this context "autonomy" means not only my right to order myself but also my right to order someone else who is in my employ to do my autonomous bidding. I also have the right to delegate my authority. My autonomy becomes someone else's heteronomy; it becomes my right to command someone else (the *heteros* or "other" in heteronomy). Thus, I authorize the physician to treat my body (as hospital consent forms make clear legally). The physician is very much my agent. (Interestingly enough, in our society a lawyer in my employ is still primarily an "officer of the court" before he or she is my agent or advocate. Thus, I have greater authority over my physician to do my bidding than I have over my lawyer, even though in the past a physician was considered to be more answerable to higher authority than a lawyer.) Carrying this logic further, I could sue a physician who did not carry out my autonomous orders. Based on that possibility, my physician might be afraid (in the sense of fear of legal consequences) to refrain from doing my bidding (perhaps even fearing loss of his or her medical license) by refusing to comply with my explicit order to end my life for me. Because that fear represents a distinct possibility, my "request" for assistance from my physician in committing suicide appears to have more authoritative power over his or her actions than would be the case if I were to request assistance in committing suicide from a family member or a friend, for example. Unlike my relationship with my physician, my relationship with my family or my friends is not (yet) governed by the law of agency.

THE PHYSICIAN ORDERS THE PATIENT
TO COMMIT SUICIDE

In the third scenario, the physician prescribes suicide or orders the patient to commit suicide. Before I explore this specific situation, however, I first consider the moral problem involved when anyone tells somebody else to commit suicide. That discussion puts the question this scenario raises into a larger context. This problem arises in a famous story in the Talmud about the martyrdom of Rabbi Hanina ben Teradyon.[31]

During the Hadrianic persecution of the Jews around the time of the failed revolt against Rome led by Bar Kokhba in the second century CE, Roman officials in the land of Israel outlawed public teaching of the Torah—probably because they suspected that the rabbis, several of whom supported Bar Kokhba's revolt, were using these public occasions to give theological warrants to Jews to join in the revolt. Several prominent rabbis of that generation, however, defied the Roman ban and risked their lives by expounding the Torah to large public gatherings. For them the religious and cultural survival of the Jewish people, which they believed depended on their continuing to teach Torah to the masses, outweighed concerns for their own physical safety.[32] One of these prominent rabbis was Rabbi Hanina ben Teradyon, who was caught by the Romans and burned at the stake. To increase his agony, the Romans placed wet tufts of wool over his heart so that "his life-breathe [*nishmato*] would not go out quickly."[33] In deep sympathy with their teacher's plight, the rabbi's disciples (who obviously were being forced to watch this spectacle, probably to strike terror in their hearts) said to him, "Rabbi! Open your mouth and let the fire enter!" In other words, they were telling him to end his life more quickly and thus end his death-agony more quickly, contrary to what the Roman murderers had planned for him. In fact, if he could do this, he would be defying the Romans in death—as he had defied them in life by publicly teaching Torah—by ending his great pain on his own terms. Yet despite great temptation, Rabbi Hanina states the most theologically compelling reason for not doing what his disciples told him to do: "It is better [*mutav*] that the One who takes it [my life] be the One who gave it [*she-natnah*], but he [a human] is not to destroy his own life himself [*ve'al yehabbel b'atsmo*]."[34] Rabbi Hanina exposed himself to death by defying the Roman proscription of publicly teaching Torah. He surely knew that this choice probably would result in his own martyrdom. Yet one great difference between a suicide and a martyr is that a person who commits suicide directly intends his or her own death; a martyr does not.[35] Unlike a person committing suicide, Rabbi Hanina did not want to die. He wanted to live and sanctify God's name in public by teaching God's Torah in public, although he was fully aware of the great danger this choice involved.

Perhaps the key to understanding Rabbi Hanina's dictum is to explain what one means when one says that God gives life. To say that this means our lives are not our possessions to destroy at will but that all lives belong to God as their creator is to beg the question.[36] Yet that assertion cannot explain why we are allowed to destroy other creatures or possessions of God when that is in our best positive interest. Indeed, humans could not survive if they were prohibited from destroying any life; the only proviso is that they do not destroy anything for the sake of destruction per se.[37] In this case, Rabbi Hanina's best interest was to end his agony in the most immediate way possible; had he done so, surely no one would blame him for it afterward. Of course, Rabbi Hanina also could have said that no creature is to destroy any human created in the image of God, and that concept would have been a good reason for not following his disciples' directive to him.[38] Humans have a different relationship with their Creator than do other creatures; therefore, human lives are inviolable in a way the lives of other creatures are not. Rabbi Hannina was making a different (although not contradictory) point to his disciples, however.

What do we mean when we say that God gives human life? To whom does God give human life? First, our lives are given to us in the sense that we are to preserve them and care for them.[39] Accordingly, no one is allowed to destroy himself or herself in the sense of forcing his or her own breath to become extinguished—which would have been the case if Rabbi Hanina had breathed in the flames as his disciples suggested. The rabbinic term "his breath expired" (*yats'ah nismato*) is the same as the Old English phrase "give up the ghost."[40] There is solid scriptural support for the position that God alone has the right to take back the breath of any of his human creatures because God alone directly gave it or placed it in the human body.[41]

We also could say that God gives our lives to persons who are charged to care for them. These persons are not authorized to harm or destroy what has been given or entrusted into their care. Thus, Rabbi Hanina's life is given to the Romans, who have political authority over him. Instead of properly keeping their charge over him, however, they chose to violate it by killing him for exercising his God-given right to teach Torah to the Jewish masses. Because their orders are illegitimate, Rabbi Hanina cannot in good conscience cooperate with them. His disciples—who, contrary to the Roman officials, are acting with the best of intentions—nonetheless have one thing in common with these officials. They have some advantage, if not literal authority, over their teacher because they are not being burned at the stake. Apparently the Roman officials allowed the rabbi's disciples to aid their teacher to have a more easy death; there is no mention that they were punished for that assistance.[42] In fact, the Roman official charged with killing Rabbi Hanina does shorten his death-agony, which seems to have been his right. Moreover, Rabbi Hanina does not suggest to himself that he end his own life. That suggestion comes from others—his disciples. He has the choice of whether to listen to them or not. As their teacher, he offers one last lesson to them regarding why he could not listen to them on this occasion.[43]

The point in this interpretation of the story of Rabbi Hanina ben Teradyon's martyrdom is that someone who has political power or authority over some other human or humans has no right to destroy or command others to destroy that human life, even if that "other" is the victim himself or herself. Any human being placed under their power is only given to their charge for care. Only the Giver of the gift can take back what He has given; the recipient of the gift, whose charge is to care for it, is not allowed to hand back the gift or cause the gift to be handed back to the Giver. Persons who are to be the objects of this care are to cooperate with their caregivers in the same way they are to resist people who are intent upon their destruction. (Recall how many prisoners in Auschwitz and other death camps refused to cooperate with the Nazis who were intent on killing them and destroying their desire to live before actually killing them.)[44]

Following the implication of Rabbi Hanina ben Teradyon's answer to his disciples, we can better understand why a physician has no right to order somebody to kill himself or herself and why the patient who receives such immoral orders has a duty to resist them.

In current parlance, "prescription" and "order" are used more often in medical contexts than in their original legal contexts: We speak of a medical prescription or doctor's orders. This transposition simply indicates, however, that the authority we have always seen in the law is increasingly taken to be a medical prerogative. To be sure, most advocates of physician-assisted suicide would insist that the patient is still autonomous even in this scenario, in the sense that the patient initially authorized the physician to treat him or her and in the sense that the patient still has the right to refuse to follow the physician's prescription at any point in their relationship. (Indeed, the patient might have chosen his or her physician because the patient knows that this physician is wont to prescribe suicide—as with patients who have sought out the prescriptions of Dr. Jack Kevorkian.) Nevertheless, because of the belief that the physician's medical expertise extends into his or her moral expertise as well, more and more patients are likely to follow their doctors' orders, believing themselves unqualified to refuse what they have been ordered to do by a medical authority.

Nevertheless, if the doctor's orders are immoral, the doctor is guilty of a sin, even though he or she is not legally punishable (in this world, anyway). Moreover, if the patient who actually commits the suicidal act does so under what we might call moral duress, the patient is less guilty, and the one who pressured this patient to commit suicide seems to be more guilty of a crime.[45] Again, we can base this judgment on Abravanel's distinction between an unofficial request from one layperson to another to commit a sin and an official order to commit a sin from one politically powerful person to another person who is under his or her power. Because the physician did not actually commit homicide (as the physician did in the first scenario and as the nurse did in the second scenario), however, what is his or her sin in prescribing suicide?

This physician probably has violated the scriptural prohibition, "You shall not place a stumbling-block [*mikhshol*] before the blind" (Leviticus 19:14). In the rabbinic tradition, this verse is not interpreted to be a prohibition of literally causing physical harm to an unsuspecting person. Instead, in the words of the oldest midrash on Leviticus, the prohibition means, "Do not give someone practical advice [*eitsah*] that is unsuitable [*sh'einah hogenet*] for him [to do]."46 Taken by itself, this reformulation of the scriptural commandment might apply only to the fourth scenario, in which the physician merely provides the patient with the means to commit suicide. Nevertheless, Maimonides, in one of his many discussions of this prohibition, writes:

> It is our principle that "there is no agency for sin" [*ein sheliah li-dvar aveirah*], and the one who actually commits the sin himself, he is the one whom the court punishes. But the one who deceives him, thus bringing him to stumble, or the one who commands him to sin [*she-tsivahu al he'aveirah*], or the one who aides him [*she-sayyeu*] in any way, even with a casual comment [*be-dibbur met*]: he is punished by God [*bi-yedei shamayim*] according to the value of what he did. . . . Nevertheless, this person is not liable for any of the punishments prescribed in the Torah; instead, he has violated what God said: "You shall not place a stumbling-block before the blind" [that is] if he enabled [*garam*] the sin to take place. Or, he has violated God's word: "Do not put your hand with the wicked" (Exodus 23:1).47

In this packed comment, Maimonides has brought together the following principles: There is no agency for sin; a sinner is not to be aided;48 anything less than full and direct causation of a forbidden act is not humanly punishable; violation of a prohibition [*l'av*]; and when no tangible act [*ma'aseh*] has occurred, is not humanly punishable.49 These four principles determine how the following two scriptural norms are to be applied: Do not enable sin to occur (Leviticus 19:14) and do not cooperate in the commission of any sin (Exodus 23:1). Moreover, by mentioning that divine punishment is according to "the value [*erekh*] of what he did," Maimonides seems to be saying that there is a difference in terms of how much or how little the one who offered the bad advice or admonition actually contributed to the act committed by the person he or she advised or admonished.

Maimonides includes among the persons who commit these sins the one who commands or prescribes someone else to sin.[50] In the present case, the one so commanded or prescribed is the patient whose suicide has been ordered by his or her physician. Anyone who entices someone else to sin, whether by mere suggestion or direct command, is put into the same category of enablers (*gormim*).[51] Yet when we again use Abravanel's phenomenological distinction between an official prescription and an unofficial request, we might be able to distinguish—morally, if not legally—between the physician who prescribes suicide and the physician who only makes the means for suicide available to his or her patient (the fourth scenario). This distinction does not exonerate the latter physician by distinguishing him or her from the much more serious offense of the suicide-prescribing physician; it is meant to show that despite the specific difference between these two types of physicians, they both have violated the same general norm or norms. The difference is that the suicide-prescribing physician has violated these norms in a more serious way than the physician who only suggests to a patient how to commit suicide. Yet the physician who only suggests suicide to his or her patient is still—in the words of Maimonides elsewhere—the "middleman" (*sirsur*) between the perpetuator of the crime and the victim of the crime, even though they are the same person.[52]

THE PHYSICIAN PREPARES THE PATIENT FOR SUICIDE

The fourth scenario and the fifth scenario are almost identical, with one significant difference. In the fourth scenario, the patient apparently would be unable to commit suicide without the specific intervention of the physician. In the fifth scenario, however, involvement by the physician seems to be less necessary for the fatal outcome; the physician simply warns the patient about the lethal effects of taking an overdose of medication. As several medieval exegetes note in commenting on the chief discussion of the prohibition of placing a stumbling-block before the blind, one could say that this prohibition has been clearly violated only when the actual perpetuator of the sin could not have gotten the means for committing the sin except from the person "placing this particular stumbling-block before him."[53]

Nevertheless, the essential question at stake in the fifth scenario is the following: What is the real intention of the physician who is offering this information? Is the physician intending to advise a patient of a possible danger to his or her life because the physician surmises that this patient will exercise care to preserve his or her life, or is the physician intending to advise the patient because the physician surmises that the patient wants to learn more precisely from his or her physician how to end his or her life? In other words, is this advice a warning or an enticement? Is it for the sake of life or death?

Clearly this question can be answered only by the physician—and by God, who "sees the heart" (I Samuel 16:7). Indeed, the oldest midrash on Leviticus states that this is why the full version of Leviticus 19:14 reads, "You shall not curse the deaf, or place a stumbling-block before the blind, but you shall fear your God, I am the Lord." The last clause makes the moral quality of the act itself a matter of the heart (*masur le-lev*), which is invisible to anyone other than the perpetuator of the act and the God he or she is either obeying or defying by this act.[54] In other words, you shall fear God, who knows what your true intention is before you commit the prohibited act and is the same God who knows what your true intention was after you commit the act and therefore can punish it properly. Thus, one should initially avoid acting out a bad intention because of respect for God's command not to harm any of God's human creatures especially, and one should subsequently fear God's punishment if one acts out his or her evil intention. Optimally, one should not commit the sin because the prohibited act is offensive to God, who prohibited it—the same God before whom one is to be always in awe—rather than out of fear of divine punishment.[55] Nevertheless, the moral quality of the act (if not its theological quality) is the same whether the act is done for the higher motive (respect for God) or the lower motive (fear of God's punishment).

This decision about whether to commit the act is strictly between God and the individual person. Moreover, in this scenario, not only can malevolent physicians escape human detection and punishment, they can even escape human opprobrium by arguing, in case of subsequent criticism, that they were only warning the patient and did not intend that the patient use this warning for a lethal purpose. Yet even if the physician is confident that his or her intention was not to help the patient end his or her life, any doubt about what the patient will do with this kind of information should give the physician considerable pause.[56] The physician should regard this doubtful situation to be "a time to be silent" rather than "a time to speak" (Ecclesiastes 3:7).[57]

Similarly when a patient requests a narcotic drug such as morphine because of his or her unbearable pain, and the physician complies with this request by prescribing such strong pain medication. A patient has the right to demand that he or she receive the most effective pain medication available, even if prolonged use of such medication might shorten his or her life. The first obligation of the physician is to care for the patient by treating the patient's unbearable pain, even if that care might make a cure for this patient's essential malady more remote or preclude it altogether.[58] (Philosophers call this situation a "double effect.")[59] The physician still must decide, however, whether his or her intention is to relieve the patient of pain, even if the patient's life will be shortened as an unintended side effect of taking pain medication, or to kill the patient (whether the patient wants to die or not) through a medical subterfuge. Although others sometimes can detect the physician's most likely intention from the prescribed dosage, drawing any such inferences from what was prescribed often is impossible. In such cases, the physician will have to answer to God alone.[60]

SUICIDE AS A REFLEXIVE ACT

As an act in which the subject and the object of the act are the same person, suicide cannot be simply subsumed under the prohibition of homicide. "To murder" is a transitive verb that describes an act that intends an object other than the actor. A person murders someone else. Thus, Maimonides paraphrases "Thou shalt not murder" as follows: "We have been commanded that some of us [*qtsatenu*] are not to kill some of us [*et qtsatenu*]."61 The use of the preposition *et*, which normally denotes a direct object, makes clear that the verb "to kill" (*le-harog*) intends someone other than the person who is commanded not to kill. Therefore, we must look somewhere else in scripture for a more precise prohibition of suicide. We must bear in mind the logical problem of who is acting upon whom when we use the transitive verb "to kill" intransitively or reflexively.

One place to begin this search is the following verse: "Surely be very diligent to care for [*u-shmor*] your own life [*nafshekha*]" (Deuteronomy 4:9). Similarly a few verses later (4:15): "Be very careful [*ve-nishmartem m'od*] with your own lives [*nafshoteikhem*]." With regard to the first verse, the Talmud tells a story about a certain pious man (*hasid*) who refuses to interrupt his prayer to return the greeting of a gentile official.62 The gentile official (*sar*) berates this man for violating the Torah's commandment to watch over his own life. After all, this official could easily kill the man for the gross insult to such an authoritative person as himself. (Significantly, the Talmud agrees with this official because in the legal context in which this story is related one should even interrupt prayer if such an interruption is required to save oneself from imminent danger to his or her own life.)63 In another place in the Talmud, this verse is interpreted as denoting a negative commandment—a "thou shalt not."64 Hence, people who do not watch over their own lives have violated this negative commandment. Surely one who is about to commit suicide is not watching over his or her own life. Again, however, the imminent danger one is to avoid is the danger to oneself from someone else. Hence, one can only vaguely infer from this commandment that one is not to endanger his or her own life when that danger to one's life comes from oneself. The self-endangering person is not fleeing the danger but pursuing it.

Moreover, harming oneself is not the simple inverse of taking care of oneself. Taking care of oneself need not involve any bifurcation of the self. When I take care of myself—eating properly and getting enough rest, for example—my body is not an object that my "self" is caring for. My body is simply exercising its own/my own natural drive to survive and live well. My mind is the part of my body that learns how to do this well, to extend and improve my life as a whole. Harming myself (of which killing myself is the most egregious example) is essentially different. It entails a bifurcation of body and mind insofar as my mind is now acting against my body by ordering one part of my body (such as my feet) to destroy my whole life (by jumping off a cliff, for example). Left to its own devices, my self would simply act for the sake of surviving and living as well as it can. When I am contemplating suicide, then, my mind becomes my self and acts against my body as a negative "other"— even if that "other" is regarded as my property or possession, which now stands opposed to my real self.

In the type of contemplated suicide for which a patient seeks a physician's assistance (such as cases in which the patient faces a future that seems to be full of further pain and debilitation), the suicidal person usually seems to want to be finished with a body with which he or she could once identify. That body had once served the patient's conscious need to live well, but now it seems to be the patient's worst enemy. In other words, if the patient's body is now acting against him or her, the patient will act against his or her body by eliminating it. One could almost say that such a suicide entails someone taking revenge on the patient's body for having deserted the patient when he or she needed it to continue to live well.

Suicide poses the logical problem of all reflexive action: Who is acting upon whom?[65] In this case, who is killing whom? Is bifurcating myself in this way not delusional, just as we would regard self-punishment as delusional? How can I be both the subject and the object of the same act? This is different when I act *for* myself such as when I feed myself. Here my body is now taking something external to itself into itself; hence the ingested food is the object I, the subject, am acting upon. But when I act *against* myself, I am externalizing my own body *from* myself, thus turning part of myself into something *apart* from me. As such, perhaps a person who is rational enough to think about committing suicide, rather than doing it spontaneously, is violating the norm, "You shall move far from what is a lie [*mi-dvar sheqer*]" (Exodus 23:7).[66] One could paraphrase this norm as follows: Do not engage in delusional thinking. Is thinking that one can transcend one's own body not delusional? Perhaps someone who is counseling a person who is contemplating suicide should help this person explore his or her thoughts to see how they stand up to rational enquiry. Of course, this exploration depends on whether this person is willing or able emotionally to engage in rational discourse.[67]

We also must carefully distinguish between suicidal patients who are suffering from clinical depression and need therapeutic intervention and patients who do not seem to be as desperately irrational in facing their own death and might need more discursive counseling. Suicidally depressed patients often want to end their own lives because of their past, which they think makes them unworthy of any more life in the present and the future. For such persons, suicide often means expiation. Because of their present perception of their past, they think they do not deserve a future. Persons who seek a physician for assistance in committing suicide, however, often want to end their lives not because they think themselves to be unworthy of a future but because they think their future will be "against" them, in contrast to a past that they think was "for" them. They do not want their future, and they cannot retrieve their past, so they want to end their present—their presence in the world.

Obviously, counseling a person who is contemplating suicide because of that person's perception of his or her future rather than his or her past (as with suicidally depressed patients) will be more effective if that person can trust the counselor to be genuinely concerned that the patient live and not die. (I return to this point when I deal with the question of how much one's desire to live or die depends on the desire of significant others in one's life regarding whether one should live or die.)

I have looked at the texts concerning self-care as distinguished from self-harm to better appreciate the Talmud's most explicit discussion of suicide, which is located in a discussion of the more specific question of self-injury—that is, injuring one's own body. Consideration of these texts provides a phenomenological perspective on the question of reflexive action that can serve as a good introduction to the following text from the Mishnah: "A person who injures himself [*ha-hovel b'atsmo*], even though not permitted to do so [*eino rash'ai*], is nonetheless exempt from legal penalty [*patur*]."⁶⁸ The Talmud discusses this text as follows: "Who was it who said 'a person is not permitted to injure himself'? One could say that it was Rabbi Eleazar, who interpreted the verse 'Your lifeblood I shall surely requite' (Genesis 9:5) to mean: From your life I shall requite your blood."⁶⁹ The Talmud quickly notes, however, that suicide may not be the same as self-injury. That is true, inasmuch as one survives harming oneself and could even think one might have to somehow "make it up" to oneself. Obviously, that would not be the case with a successful suicide. In the case of suicide, there is no time afterward—at least in any place of which we are currently aware.⁷⁰

In a case of less-than-fatal self-injury, one survives one's past act by living one's life in the present, and one can look back on that past apart from one's present self. One's past action becomes one's present memory of an experience: What one did becomes what happened to one "back then." One is now responsible for having injured oneself. Hence, one has a future in which one could act differently than one did in the past, learning in the present from one's past mistake. The Jewish tradition calls such regretful learning from one's past mistakes "repentance" (*teshuvah*).⁷¹

With no future in which to act in this world, however, a person who commits suicide has no opportunity for any such remorse in this world of mortal beings. One's responsibility for a suicide committed in this world will be judged by God in the world to come; with regard to the judgment for any questionable act committed in this world, God alone knows the heart and its true motives and will surely judge whether the successful suicide was compelled by forces beyond one's control to stop them or not. (In this world, however, we judge all suicides after the fact as having been compelled by forces beyond the person's control, and that judgment should include persons who seemingly commit suicide as the result of a contemplated, deliberate choice.)

This analysis is evident in Rabbi Eleazar's exegesis of Genesis 9:5, which implies that Rabbi Eleazar is not giving the *prima facie* meaning (or *peshat*) of this verse. Taken by itself and in its own immediate context, the verse translates literally as follows: "Surely I shall require [*edrosh*] your life-blood [*et dimekhem le-nafshoteikhem*] from the hand of every beast I shall require it, and from the hand of a man's brother I shall require the life of that person [*ha'adam*]." In other words, the scripture is talking about God punishing anyone who kills another human being.[72] As the succeeding verse (Genesis 9:6) explains in justifying human beings helping God's execution of justice for other human beings (on occasions when they can do so by participating in divine justice), that is "because [*ki*] He made humans in the image of God [*tselem elohim*]." God has a special concern for justice being done to or for human creatures created in God's image. One may be reminded of what God said to Cain after he had murdered Abel—"The voice of your brother's blood is crying to me from the ground" (Genesis 4:10)—and how Cain begged not to be put in a position whereby "whoever finds me will kill me" (Genesis 4:14)—that is, with impunity.

Rabbi Eleazar's exegesis, however, has turned what seems to be a transitive relationship between the killer and his victim and between the killer and the God of justice into an intransitive, reflexive relationship between two parts of one self. That is, one's life-blood is now bifurcated into two opposing parties: one's life or self and one's blood or body.[73] The question is whether one can really accomplish that bifurcation successfully. Can one really transcend one's own bodily existence, one's own natural embodiment (with suicide the most radical self-bifurcation possible)? The reemphasis of God's judgment on the person who attempts to bifurcate himself or herself so radically, so ultimately, is meant to suggest that this most radical attempt at transcendence of one's embodied self will be brought to final defeat by God. One's self-immolation will come to naught: One will still die within the agony of one's own life; indeed, it might be one's greatest agony. Without the transcendence of a future, one will never escape one's present predicament.

This line of thinking might explain a traditional Jewish teaching regarding suicide: "One who kills himself willingly [*ha-me'abed atsmo le-da'at*] has no portion in the world to come." Although this principle sounds rabbinic, several scholars have noted that they could not find a literary source for this teaching anywhere in the Babylonian or Palestinian Talmud or in any of the Midrashim.[74] I am not suggesting that Rabbi Eleazar's exegesis of Genesis 9:5 is the textual source of this teaching—only that the concept his exegesis implies can be connected to this teaching. That is, this teaching seems to be speaking against a Jew who might think (along the lines of the Stoics) that ending his or her life in this world will release his or her soul from the agony of this world for the ecstasy or bodily transcendence of the world to come.[75] This notion of self-transcendence is encouraged by the idea that the soul (*nefesh*) is a substance that is separate from the body and therefore can survive into the future without the body. That type of anthropology appears to be at odds with scriptural teaching, however.[76]

One could make a good case that in scripture, the word *nefesh*, usually translated as "soul," in fact means the capacity of an animal body for locomotion and communication beyond bodily touching—especially hearing, speaking, and seeing. That interpretation might explain that the most definite rabbinic teaching about the world to come is the doctrine of the resurrection of the dead (*tehiyyat ha-metim*), which clearly means resurrection of the body to an everlasting existence at the end of days (*ahareet ha-yamim*).[77] If one regards the Christian doctrine of the resurrection of the dead as an appropriation of the Jewish (specifically pharisaic-rabbinic) doctrine of the resurrection of the dead, an insight of the great Christian theologian Reinhold Niebuhr (d. 1991) is apt in this context: "[T]he resurrection of the body is . . . both more individual and more social in its connotations than the more alternative idea of the immortality of the soul . . . because it asserts eternal significance, not for some impersonal *nous* which has no real relation to the actual self; but for the self as it exists in the body."[78] Indeed, the doctrine of resurrection of the human body emphasizes the impossibility of humans ever permanently transcending the embodied nature they share with all the other animals (*nefashot*) God has created, in this world or for the next.[79]

SUICIDE AND PERSONAL RESPONSIBILITY

The major logical problem involved in positing reflexive action is that the subject and the object of the act are identical, yet in ordinary reality nothing can both be and not be the same thing at the same time. In practical terms, this problem again raises the question: Who is acting upon whom? This logical and ethical paradox was best expressed by Plato, who wrote, "Now the phrase 'master of himself' [*hauton*] is an absurdity, is it not? For he who is master of himself would also be subject to himself, and he who is subject to himself would be master . . . the same person [*ho autos*]."[80]

Plato's solution to this problem is to divide the soul into a better part and a worse part; he advocates that the better part rule the worse part rather than vice versa. Yet Plato avoids the problem of self-bifurcation that is evident in the delusional thinking of persons who are contemplating suicide. Plato does not regard this conflict within the soul as primarily an internal relation. Instead, one could say that Plato sees each of these two parts of the soul intending a reality that transcends it but to which it is still related. Thus, the worse part of the soul is related to the physical world through appetite, whereas the better part of the soul is related to the world of the eternal, intelligible Forms (at the apex of which is the Good itself) through intellect (*nous*).

Moreover, the intelligible world is not intelligible because I know it; I know it because it is intelligible.[81] Similarly, the physical world is not desirable because I desire it; I desire it because it is desirable. These two external realities have always been before me, and they will still be there after their brief encounter within my soul. The human soul, as it were, is merely one arena where the intelligible world and the physical world first collide and then, optimally, work out an arrangement so that intelligence both directs and cares for bodily appetite in a way that bodily appetite could not possibly care for itself.[82]

I bring this analysis into the discussion of the moral problem of physician-assisted suicide because by referring the part of oneself that one considers to be one's higher or true self to an external, higher, truer reality and then seeing that reality as the true origin of one's existentially significant acts—among which suicide certainly belongs—one thereby places ultimate responsibility for these acts beyond and above oneself. Consider how one places oneself under what one believes is the benevolent authority of one's physician. When one places primary responsibility for one's acts in physical or psychic forces outside of oneself or one's consciousness or beyond one's will, one need only admit to the secondary responsibility of freely cooperating with them. If one feels that one could not have done otherwise, one need take no responsibility for one's acts because one has thereby demoted their moral character to that of behavior.

If I believe myself to be under the orders of someone who is greater than myself in power and wisdom, I can avoid ultimate responsibility for my act against myself by asserting that it is really the other who acted through me, using my will to accomplish his or her purposes—in this case elimination of the body that is mine but not me. Why did I follow these orders? I believed that other was acting through me for my welfare—that he or she knows what is best for me better than I do myself and that he or she has far greater power to affect my welfare than I have.[83] Therefore, even if that authority commands me to do something that seems to be against myself, such as killing myself, I justify this command by saying to myself (and others) that my body is no longer serving my true self; it is hindering my full functioning or flourishing in this world, so I need to get rid of it. The other has authorized me to do just that. As such, I am saved from the moral dilemma of self-destruction because my true self is not eliminated, nor does my true self originate the elimination of this troublesome bodily possession.

By using this kind of thinking—which seems more rational than the more radical autonomy I discuss above—I am more easily exonerated from primary responsibility for my seemingly destructive act because although my act was freely chosen, it was not autonomous.[84] It was a response to the command of an authority that was already there before I made my choice. Thus, although I am exonerated from the primary responsibility of autonomy, I still have the secondary responsibility of freedom inasmuch as that higher authority can impose his or her moral authority over me only when I accept his or her authority freely, based on what I know about the difference between what is good or bad for me. At a minimum, I know what is bad for me, so I would not accept that authority if he or she were advocating through me something that is evidently bad for me. That is so however little I know what is good for me and however little power I have to effect what is good for me. Furthermore, this external factor is not just acting upon me transitively; it is acting with my cooperation. Thus, our relationship is a transaction; it is much more than the power of an active cause over a passive effect.

Theologically speaking, when the Torah commands one to do something good for somebody else, one should regard oneself as cooperating with God's beneficence in the world. The subject of the commandment (*metsuveh*) is the person who is commanded to benefit the other person, who is the object of the commandment; God, however, is both the source of the commandment and its ultimate end. If the subject of the commandment takes primary responsibility for the good that has been done through him or her, that person is guilty of self-righteousness or moral exhibitionism (*yohara*).[85] This self-righteousness is clearly out of order because the true intent of the person so commanded is to direct attention to the human object of the commandment and the divine source of the commandment, especially when the deed is being done as an act of *imitatio Dei*.[86] This ascription of primary responsibility away from oneself is not appropriate, however, when one is the subject of an act that is designed to harm another person.

When one harms another person (or oneself, as in the case of suicide), even though we assume that God's will was that this other person be harmed, we cannot infer from that assumption that God actually willed this harm to be effected by this particular person.[87] We only know (as distinct from assuming) what God's will is from what we have been commanded to do in the Torah. When one is doing harm to somebody else, one cannot ascribe primary responsibility to God away from oneself because God did not command one to do this harm to anybody. (Even human punishment of criminals is considered to have been commanded for their benefit, as well as for the benefit of their victims—that is, criminals benefit from the punishment that ultimately takes their criminality.)[88] Therefore, the intention of the person doing harm could only be the exercise of his or her own primary, autonomous responsibility.

Thus, when one submits oneself to the authority of someone one knows to be illegitimate, one cannot ascribe primary responsibility for one's act to that person (whether individual or collective) away from oneself.

Indeed, such evasion of primary responsibility was what Adam and Eve attempted when they disobeyed God in the Garden of Eden, even though they knew better. Each of them claimed to be only an accomplice: Adam blamed Eve, and Eve blamed the serpent who first promised them autonomy when he said, "You will become like God" (Genesis 3:5). Adam and Eve wanted autonomy when they were tempted by the egocentricity it promised, but they disclaimed it when they saw the undesired judgment that came because of its exercise. Rather than giving them power over the world, the exercise of their autonomy brought them into the world and made them dependent on its natural processes by making them conscious of their mortality.[89]

The desire to attribute ultimate responsibility elsewhere, even for acts one could do for oneself, appears in a little-noticed insight of Maimonides. Suggesting a rationale for denial of self-incrimination as a sufficient reason for punishing a self-incriminator, he writes:

Scripture decrees that a court does not execute anyone . . . by his own testimony [*be-hotsa'at peev*], but only by the testimony of two witnesses. . . . the Sanhedrin is not to execute or physically punish anyone who admits [*ha-modeh*] to a sin since he may have lost his mind [*shema nitrafah da'ato*] in this matter. Perhaps he is one of those wretched, bitter-spirited [*marei nefesh*] people who long for death by plunging swords into their bellies or who throw themselves off roofs. So perhaps this is the case with this one: he says [that is, he confesses to] something he did not do in order to be killed [*kedei she-yehareg*].[90]

In this passage, which is taken from Maimonides' larger treatment of capital punishment in his great compendium of Jewish law, Maimonides could be referring to three different types of people who are likely to incriminate themselves. He might be referring to deranged persons who confess to crimes they did not commit but actually believe they did commit. (Today, for example, when a sensational murder has been committed, deranged persons often come forward and confess to police that they are the criminals and deserve full punishment for their crimes.) Maimonides also might be referring to severely depressed persons, wracked with exaggerated guilt, who know they did not commit the crime but believe they deserve the same punishment as whoever did commit the crime. Finally, Maimonides might be referring to suicidal persons, who—although not seemingly wracked with guilt (imagined or real)—want to die but do not want to take primary responsibility for instigating their own death. Therefore, such persons will do anything to make their own death an execution by someone else and thus the primary responsibility of a higher other—an official with greater political authority than any individual.

In a society that does not authorize physician-assisted suicide but does convict persons who have incriminated themselves, this approach might be the only way to accomplish that type of officially approved suicide. Therefore, Maimonides regards the Torah's rejection of self-incrimination as a way of eliminating the possibility of that type of subterfuge in Jewish criminal procedures.

Maimonides' point about this danger in criminal confessions is psychological rather than legal. He is talking about the psychological motivation of the self-incriminator, not why someone does not have the legal right to incriminate oneself. To be sure, the third interpretation stretches Maimonides' text inasmuch as he specifically mentions the fact that it could be the strategy of someone who is suicidally depressed. Indeed, such persons might regard their death as some sort of expiation—and one cannot expiate oneself, for the reasons I discuss in critiquing the notion of a truly reflexive act. Thus, Maimonides' psychological point has a theological implication because, in a religious context, expiation is performed by a priest as an official designated by the religious community to rectify some sort of breach in the body politic of that community. The suicidal person wants to be relieved of his or her guilt for what he or she did against others—those others being the community itself in the person of one or several of its members, and God being the Sovereign of that community.[91]

Thus, the executioner is performing a political and theological function. Indeed, the convicted criminal believes he or she needs the ministrations of the community, through its officials, to be relieved of his or her guilt. Thus, the Mishnah states that a criminal who has been sentenced to death is to say just before he or she is put to death, "May my death be atonement [*kapparah*] for all my iniquities."[92] This preexecution confession is *post factum* self-incrimination, coming from one who has been incriminated and convicted by the testimony of others *ab initio*. In fact, the Mishnah regards such self-incrimination as a necessary prerequisite for the chastened criminal to gain the life of the world to come.[93] He or she must accept the forfeiture of his or her life in this world as just expiation. In a way, the criminal's death is a sacrifice.

Even if there is no expression of what we might call pathological guilt on the part of a person who is requesting his or her own death from someone else, is such a request to a public official—such as a physician who is licensed by the state—not intended to have that official take public responsibility for what otherwise would be the most private of acts? This question leads into the issue of the relationship of individuals to others in that society and the relationship of that society to its individual members. How does that mutual relationship work in the case of a member of the society who wants to die with the society's authorization? Indeed, this situation also might reflect a feeling of guilt, inasmuch as that person might be requesting an authorized death from the very society he or she feels so guilty about having failed.

These questions can be asked even in a secular society. As such, they can be asked in philosophical discourse about suicide and assisted suicide. That understanding leads into the philosophical consideration of the issue of physician-assisted suicide and then into some of the political implications of the philosophical reflection on this issue.

PUBLIC PHILOSOPHY IN A SECULAR SOCIETY

The foregoing discussion is largely theological inasmuch as it draws its points from a careful reading of texts from the Jewish theological tradition—that is, texts that are taken to be either revelation or the explication and elaboration of revelation. It also is theological in that it invokes issues that are inherent in the relationship between God and humans—specifically, between God and the Jewish people, who are the recipients of the revelation of the Torah. Yet that discussion also is philosophical in that it deals with how the bearers of Jewish tradition have been continually engaged in what philosophers have called practical reason, which is the reason involved in understanding interhuman relations and how they are governed by rational norms.[94] Nevertheless, the discussion takes place within the Jewish tradition—the tradition of a people for whom God is the Sovereign in the sense that He is the direct source of this people's law and the final Judge of whether this law has been kept or violated by the community and each of its members. Yet traditional Jews can engage in much of that practical reason within the public discourse of a secular society (without being disingenuous) when they are talking to others outside their own traditional community on issues such as physician-assisted suicide.

By secular society I do not mean a society in which a requirement for entrance into its public discourse is that one be a *de facto* atheist—that is, a person who agrees never to mention his or her or anyone else's relationship with God in public (even if such persons are tolerated in that they are allowed to have a private relationship with God). I cannot be a participant in that kind of public discourse if that is what is required of me and others like me, regardless of whether some secularists today would like that to be the case. Because I consider myself and others like me (from my own religion and from other religions) to be capable of entering secular public discourse in good faith, however, I have to present and argue for a more minimal requirement for entrance into that kind of public discourse.

That minimal requirement for entrance into secular public discourse is that I cannot invoke the authority of my tradition and its founding revelation and rightfully expect a hearing because of it. I may only make arguments and suggestions that are rational (and, I hope, persuasive) to my fellow participants in that discourse, regardless of whether they come from my own or another tradition of revelation (such as Christianity or Islam). Moreover, I should not be prohibited from bringing rational arguments that have been developed within my tradition, as long as I do not do so dogmatically.

I even think these arguments can mention God, as long as I do not make acceptance of God's authority, as revealed to any particular people, a precondition of that secular public discourse to be accepted by all participants in it *ab initio*. The most I can and should say about my God, if I am questioned during public discourse about my metaphysical commitments, is that I believe that the rational arguments I am making reflect the wisdom (*hokhmah*) by which God governs the universe, which He has revealed in the Torah. My arguments, then, are more my discovery than my invention. Nevertheless, I can only allude to that divine wisdom; I cannot invoke it as a premise in any public argument and expect anyone outside my own theological circle to listen.[95]

Secularists cannot require *de facto* atheism (often called by the more benign name agnosticism) on the part of religious people as a prerequisite for entrance into public discourse (which at its best is philosophical dialogue) with themselves and expect religious people to accept a precondition that causes them to be untrue to their fundamental metaphysical commitments. Similarly, religious people cannot expect secularists to acknowledge the authority of any revelation as a precondition for entrance into public discourse with religious people because doing so would require such secularists to be untrue to their fundamental metaphysical commitments.

Thus, the first requirement for the entrance of a theologian such as myself into public discourse on an issue such as physician-assisted suicide is that I must be able to argue as a philosopher without being required to deny, even implicitly, my fundamental theological or metaphysical commitments. That requirement comes from the side of philosophy. The second requirement, however, comes from the side of theology. As a traditionalist Jewish theologian, I must always be sure that the public arguments and suggestions I make as a philosopher do not contradict the normative teaching of the Jewish tradition, even if these arguments and suggestions do not always have to be drawn directly from the Jewish tradition as presented in its authoritative texts such as the Bible and the Talmud. This requirement is not difficult, however, because the Jewish tradition, in my reading, does not present norms governing interhuman relations that are inherently irrational or even nonrational.

SUICIDE: PRIVATE AND PUBLIC

The issue of physician-assisted suicide arises at an important inter-section between the realm of the private and the public. On one hand, suicide is the most private of all acts. It is what I can do with myself most radically. In most cases, I can accomplish it entirely in private, with nobody else involved. On the other hand, physician-assisted suicide is a very public act, not only because the suicide in-volves another person but even more so because that other person is someone who has official status. The physician must be officially licensed and therefore is not only the agent of the patient but also the agent or representative of the society that authorizes him or her to practice medicine in its midst. The question is whether killing myself is a subset of a more basic right of mine: the right "to be let alone" (in the memorable phrase of the great American lawyer and jurist Louis D. Brandeis).[96] Is killing myself, in fact, the greatest ex-ercise of my right to privacy? Conversely, is my right to kill myself, within my larger right to privacy, something society (through the institution of state officials) should revoke by invading my privacy, as it were, when I have abused that right by harming myself—and most likely harming the people who are nearest and dearest to me? Furthermore, do I have a duty to either kill myself directly or co-operate with a public official who orders my death because society (through its authorities) has determined that my death is in that society's best interest? Is my right to privacy virtually absolute, or is it much more conditional, contingent upon the approval of the society on which I am so dependent for my life and well-being in this world?

One might consider this issue within the more general ques-tions: What do I owe society; what does society owe me, and what if these duties are at odds with one another? What is the essential relation between the individual, private person and his or her soci-ety? Does the public realm derive its authority from the private realm—for example, through a social contract, which presupposes that the parties are extending their experience of private, one-on-one agreements to the larger realm of the one and the many? Or does the private realm have to recede before the authority of the public realm whenever it seems to be working against the public interest or common good because the public realm is prior to it both in time and in authority? With regard to physician-assisted suicide, is the physician primarily the agent of the patient who engages him or her or of the society that authorizes him or her to practice medicine?

A recent form of modern liberalism greatly diverges from the views of most philosophers from Plato through at least Kant. For the sake of distinction, I call this latter view classical. More recent liberalism has designated privacy as the foundation of all rights and duties. The radically individualistic claims for privacy that some contemporary liberals make rest on the idea of an autonomy that is more radically conceived than ever before.[97] Their view goes far beyond what even Kant, the most prominent advocate of autonomy in western philosophy, advocated. Kant accepted the correlation of moral rights and moral duties. In fact, he gave moral duties priority over moral rights. He did so on the basis of his acceptance of the classical idea of human nature and its essential sociality. Kant required the exercise of autonomy to be universalizable—that is, an act that everyone else in a similar situation ought to do; an act that treats the actor and all others like him or her as ends in themselves; and an act by a member of a society of similarly autonomous persons.[98] For Kant, anything that did not fulfill these three conditions was not autonomy but licentiousness.

In the type of foundational autonomy that locates itself in the exercise of my right to privacy, I am my own creator, and I am the creator of a realm in which I am the only member. Such autonomy is more narcissism than solipsism because I very much want others to recognize my autonomy by respecting it in their attitudes and in their deeds toward me. Nonetheless, at the core of my existence I am alone. My privacy is myself. Everyone else is a stranger, whose recognition of my own autonomy I crave—but only when it suits my physical or economic interests. When I need not pursue these interests, however, I gladly return to my private world. In this view, my public involvement is a necessary evil. Its value is purely instrumental. Public responsibility is merely a limit on my autonomous action that I am willing to negotiate with society in return for a nonaggression pact among all the members of society, myself included. In effect, it is a compromise: I accept limits on the projection of my autonomy in return for the society's protection against persons who would deprive me of my autonomy and its fruits. (To be politically effective, such compliance with the basic terms of the social contract is required of everyone who wants to reside within this society's jurisdiction.) The state is the institution we create to make sure that no one can cheat on this compromise, this social contract, with impunity.

Because such private, selfish persons cannot expect any trust from one another or any true loyalty from either side, however, they cannot constitute a true community among themselves. Instead, they must create the state as an external institution (heteronomy) that stands above and against its citizens in their autonomous privacy. The state is like a policeman who stands over and against potential criminals to frighten them into obeying the law. According to this metaphor, because no one really desires the authority of the state and everyone simply puts up with it in the face of the greater evil of anarchy, everyone in society is a potential criminal, hoping to cheat the authority of the state without bringing society down in the process (thus distinguishing a private criminal from, for example, a "public enemy" or a terrorist). In this view, nobody could be a hero because no one would sacrifice himself or herself for a society that no one could possibly love.

Furthermore, because such societies have a way of developing institutional interests of their own, the citizens they regulate quickly develop as much distrust of this alien, external, governmental institution as they have for each other as potentially dangerous strangers. That is why so many people put undue trust in the courts, believing that an independent judiciary will protect them when the state would deprive them of their autonomy and its fruits. Yet that judiciary frequently becomes independent not only of the power of the state but also of the citizenry by developing its own institutional interests. Thus, the judiciary also becomes a stranger to the people of its society—and sometimes even their enemy.

With the philosophical emphasis on foundational privacy, which has become more and more the norm in U.S. and Canadian courts, there can be no return to any legal prohibition of suicide. Such a prohibition would now be regarded as an unwarranted invasion of this foundational privacy.[99] This foundational privacy also would be the reason the relationship between a person and his or her physician increasingly is regarded as a private contract—an agreement between a consumer and a service provider. As long as that private contract is not a conspiracy to harm a third party, the contract can even be a suicide pact wherein the patient delegates his or her physician to kill him or her, with or without any specific conditions.

Whereas suicide involves a one-party relationship with oneself (albeit a relationship that requires a radical bifurcation of what we normally take to be the unity of body and soul), physician-assisted suicide involves a two-party relationship between the suicidal patient and his or her physician. Is this two-party relationship all there is to it, however? Does the state enter into this relationship as a third party? If so, where does the state enter the relationship? May the state enter only at the behest of one of the parties claiming the contract has been breached by the other party? Alternatively, does the state itself create the relationship of patient and physician, and does it therefore have prior rights over the relationship itself and both of the two parties thereto?

Following the "libertarian" view of foundational privacy as radical autonomy, one would have to say that the state has no business in the two-party contract that the parties have worked out by themselves (or through their lawyers), for themselves. Indeed, the only business the state would have is to be available, through the police and the courts, to intervene when the contract has been violated and the aggrieved party claims the assistance of the state to rectify the wrong done to him or her. This would be the case, for example, if a physician wants to sue his or her patient in court for nonpayment of an agreed upon fee. It also would be the case if a suicidal patient wants to sue his or her physician for being unsuccessful in killing him or her, whether deliberately or through ineptitude. The state would be functioning to effect what Aristotle called "rectifying justice" (*to diorthōtikon*).[100]

If the state interferes only when it is summoned by an individual person who believes himself or herself to have been wronged by another individual (or corporate person), most of us would regard such a minimal state as morally deficient. Most of us also expect the state to protect us, not only from each other but also from other threats to our lives and well-being. Thus, we expect the state to protect us from foreigners who would wage war against us (whether as soldiers or as terrorists) by maintaining a combat-ready military establishment, which even may be called upon to carry out preemptive strikes against highly probable enemies on their own turf. We may expect the state to protect us from natural disasters such as hurricanes and tornados by providing accurate weather forecasting, coordinated evacuation efforts, and coordinated relief from the damage these natural disasters cause to life, health, and property. We might expect the state to protect us from poverty by providing welfare and unemployment compensation if we cannot work or cannot find work. We may expect the state to protect us from ignorance by providing a system of public education. We might expect the state to provide universal health care for all citizens and residents to protect us from disease and its effects, both by preventing illness (e.g., through inoculation) and by providing treatment when we do become ill.[101]

In all of these cases, we would say that the state as the institution of society has an interest in the physical safety and economic security of its citizens, to protect them from physical and economic harm as much as possible. Accordingly, we expect the state to intervene in our privacy for the sake of "the common good" (*bonum commune*). We might define this common good to be what we expect society as a whole and its individual members to care about— namely, the physical, economic, and moral quality of their communal life together. Thus, in the event of a military threat, we expect the state to invade our privacy by drafting our young and able people into military service or putting us under surveillance if there is reason to believe we are aiding the enemy. When there is a threat of a great natural disaster, we expect the state to invade our privacy by requiring us to abandon our possessions if retaining these possessions would impede its efforts to evacuate or rescue ourselves and others. When there is widespread poverty and economic depression, we expect the state to invade our privacy by taking more of our money in taxes or curtailing benefits we conceive to be public entitlements to us as private citizens (including corporations).

Could we justify the state's invasion of the privacy of our own bodies and what we do with them? Could we justify a legal prohibition of suicide to save suicidal persons from their own self-destructive designs? In the absence of a legal prohibition of suicide, could we justify the state's invasion of one's right to contract a physician by prohibiting physicians from cooperating with the irrational designs of their suicidal patients—that is, prohibiting them from becoming their patients' self-summoned angel of death? How could we justify such an invasion of privacy—on the grounds that it is being done in the public interest or for the common good?

The question is whether privacy is foundational and the claims of the state to invade our privacy are exceptional. Conversely, are the claims of the state upon us in our privacy foundational and our privacy outside those claims exceptional?

SOCIETY'S CLAIMS ON THE INDIVIDUAL PERSON

The priority of society's claims on the individual person is well expressed by Aristotle. In his discussion of justice—the excellence that governs interpersonal relations—Aristotle mentions that justice toward oneself can be considered only in a "metaphorical and analogical sense."[102] As the discussion of the bifurcation of the self—admittedly influenced by Plato and, especially, by Aristotle—suggests, it is difficult to see how one is literally related to oneself without falling into absurdity. Aristotle's example regarding the general point he is making concerns what sort of injustice suicide is: "[T]he law does not sanction suicide (and what it does not expressly sanction, it forbids). . . . But he who kills himself voluntarily does an injury against right principle [*orthon logon*] which the law [*ho nomos*] does not allow. Therefore the suicide commits injustice [*adikei*]; but against whom? It seems to be against the state [*tēn polin*] rather than against himself [*auton*]. . . . That is why the state exacts a penalty; suicide is punished by certain marks of dishonour."[103]

The foregoing passage deals with the relationship between the individual human person and the *polis*, which is the realm of the fullest kind of human community (*koinōnia*) for Aristotle.[104] What we call the state is only the structure of this complete human community; its substance is what we call culture. Nonetheless, the laws of the *polis* are enacted and enforced by its government. That enactment, however, is for the sake of the culture of the *polis*. The culture of the society is very much concerned with what that society regards as its purpose in the world.

The notion that suicide, as the most extreme exercise of the right to privacy, is an injustice against the state strongly suggests that it violates a prior right or claim of the state. What is that right? Elsewhere Aristotle explicitly remarks that citizens belong to the state as its parts (*morion*).[105] Thus, a person who commits suicide wrongly deprives (*privare*) the state of one of its members. Suicide is a private act that deprives the state of what rightfully belongs to the state. Suicide is a citizen's desertion of the duty each person owes the state as his or her master.[106]

Yet is this assumption not the very presupposition of totalitarian regimes? Do these regimes not assume—indeed, proclaim—that human persons within their domain (including persons under their power as well as persons they plan to bring under their power) are their property? Does this assumption mean that such personal chattel of the state are to live when the state orders them to live and, for the same reason, die when the state orders them to die? Are persons not used and discarded in such societies depending on how the state perceives its needs, even when such perceptions are written into the positive law of the state and are not just the ad hoc whim of its rulers? Surely this fact, for which we need not go back to antiquity to find gruesome examples (the past century or so more than suffices for that), is the historical stimulus that has so many people so concerned with the right to privacy as the assurance of human dignity after Auschwitz and the gulag. Surely this fear is legitimate and deserves an answer before we try to make the state's claim on individual lives the basis for the prohibition of suicide and subsequent prohibition of complicity with anyone who is planning his or her own death.

Assuming that society has a claim on our lives, we clearly cannot assume an absolute prohibition of suicide—a categorical imperative—from this premise.[107] Even though in most cases society wants its members to live and not die and thus claims their lives for itself, there are times when society wants some of its members to die and thus claims their deaths for itself. This notion arises in a discussion of suicide by Plato (Aristotle's teacher): "Now he that slays the person who is, as men say, nearest and dearest of all, what penalty should he suffer? I mean the man who slays himself . . . when this is not legally ordered [*taxasēs dikē*] by the State."[108] Aristotle's readers no doubt would recall how Plato's teacher, Socrates, was sentenced to death by Athens for invoking the authority of a non-Athenian god (similar to the biblical prescription of death for the worship of "other gods") and that Socrates was required to administer the deadly dose of hemlock to himself, under official Athenian supervision.[109] That is, Socrates was duty bound to kill himself for Athens. That was the law of Athens, which Socrates himself did not consider unjust—nor did he deny the Athenian court the right to judge him according to that law, even though he believed himself to be innocent of having violated it and argued accordingly at his trial. Socrates' acceptance of what the law decreed in his case was demonstrated by his self-destruction of his own body—the body owned by the state. Socrates willingly, even cheerfully, drank the hemlock.[110]

Conceivably, following this logic, the state could require suicide from the persons it owns for other reasons as well. For example, in the case of a person contemplating suicide, could the state require a physician it licenses to urge a patient to accept his or death sentence by "autonomously" authorizing it? If a patient does not or cannot do that, could the state require (formally or informally) the physician to perform the patient's duty for him or her? This line of reasoning leads to the following question: What does the society, through its culture and its government, regard as its basic purpose, its *raison d'être*? A society's perception of its *raison d'être* will largely determine its stands on major issues of public policy. Surely the question of assisted suicide of any kind is such a major public policy issue.

If a society regards its main purpose as its own survival, physically and economically, and the overriding purpose of every member of that society as contributing to that ultimate end, persons who contribute to that end are allowed, even encouraged, to live.

Those who detract from that end, who are a drain on that society's resources or a perceived threat to them, are to be eliminated in one way or another. Following this logic, to make such useless members of society feel they are doing their proper duty to society and to make the authorities (or "statesmen") feel they are humane, should these useless people not be given the opportunity to act as if suicide really is what they would have wanted for themselves even if they had not been urged by the state to do so?

Many liberals, however, would say that is not the purpose of a society. A society's purpose is to protect the individual interests of its members. Following this logic, the state does not own its members. Of course, there is still ownership; instead of the state owning its citizens, however, the citizens of the state own themselves and, by extension, their property as well.[111] In this view of self-ownership, my self is distinguished from my body: My self is me, and my body belongs to myself; I am the master of my body, and my body is a slave of myself. As such, the state has no right to interfere in what I do with my own body, which is my property, as long as I am not harming anyone else with it (for example, killing myself by blowing up an airplane in which I am only one of many passengers).

Accordingly, an absolutist state imposes only a conditional prohibition of suicide, and a liberal state imposes none at all. Where there is no prohibition of suicide, prohibiting assisted suicide of any kind is much more difficult, except by invoking reasons that are far weaker and more tenuous than a prohibition of being an accomplice in the commission of a crime.

What if we look at a different model, however, of what the *raison d'être* of a society should be and what the *raison d'être* of its members could be? Such a model might enable us to drop the notion of ownership altogether—whether collective or individual— when we talk about the social nature of human beings and the norms presented for society's enhancement. It might enable us to ground a prohibition of suicide and a prohibition of assisting suicide, morally if not legally (a point I discuss in the next section), differently from what is grounded in the collectivist or individualist model.

What if the prime *raison d'être* of a society is to care for all of its members in ways they are not able to care for themselves by themselves? This caring can be understood in three senses:

- The state is not to harm any of its members, except when harming a member of the society is necessary to protect the society from allowing that member to harm others, as with incarceration of criminals.

- The state is to protect its members from harm from which these members cannot protect themselves—except in war, when the state must put its military personnel in harm's way.

- The state, in word and in deed, is to continually assure all of its members that the society as a whole values their continued presence, for as long as possible, except criminals whose crimes are so horrendous and so threatening to the very existence of society that no society can tolerate their presence in its midst, as in the case of high treason or terrorism.[112]

In all three of these senses of the prime *raison d'être* of the society, the society's secondary *raison d'être*—the survival of the society—is invoked only in extraordinary circumstances. Ordinarily, society is in the business of caring for its members first and foremost, and the society's interest in its own survival ordinarily does not contradict that essential purpose. Part of that care should be the society's concern for self-destructive, suicidal persons, and society should show that care by doing everything it can to save any of its members who are threatened by harm—even if that harm is self-chosen behavior, as in the case of suicide, or quasi-suicidal behavior on the part of alcoholics or drug addicts. Society also should do everything it can to prohibit or at least discourage anyone from aiding somebody else's self-destruction. Because physicians derive their authorization to function as medical practitioners in a society from that society's governmental bureaucracy, even if a society cannot formally prohibit suicide as a crime in law it can still prohibit a physician from assisting a patient in committing suicide and punish a physician who violates this prohibition, on the grounds that such assistance is contrary to the true interests of society and the true interests of the patient who makes such a request.

Does society know what the true interest of a patient is, however? What if the suicidal patient thinks that suicide is in his or her best interest? Does society know what is better for a person than that person himself or herself does? I would say yes when what a person wants is not what he or she needs.[113] For many people, of course, this line of reasoning sounds very much like the rationalizations of totalitarian regimes that claim they know what is best for their citizens (and everybody else they can lay their hands on)— even if the result is that their citizens "volunteer" for espionage or suicide missions or incarceration in a concentration camp for "reeducation" because these citizens really need to do such things for the state.

I am not speaking of needs the state invents for its citizens, however. I am speaking of human needs that the state does not invent. This type of caring entails recognizing and responding to the needs of all members of society when that society accepts this charge as its *raison d'être*. Accordingly, when a society recognizes that humans are essentially social beings, with social needs—minimally, to be alive and present to others in the world—that society must do everything it can to prevent any sort of lethal violence against anybody living in its midst, regardless of who perpetuates such violence and who the victim of such violence happens to be.

From whom does the state accept this purpose as its fundamental charge in the world? Does it not come from the members of the society who have set up and support the state in its primary function of caring for them and all others like them? How do they so charge the state? Is it not by being born into that society—by virtue of the fact that, for most of them, the state enabled their parents to marry and bring them into that society as members of one of its constituent families?[114] Family is the beginning of community, and society is an association of many communities.[115] As such, humans have a claim on the state for its care through their initial claim on their families to care for them—a claim all humans make with their first cries and tears. After expressing their need for the attention of their family from infancy on, children also need to hear from their family, in word and in deed, that their family wants them. (In fact, we know that children whose conscious social needs are not met suffer even more than children whose physical needs are not met.)

This desire for one's presence to others in the world, first in the family, should be extended into the larger community as far as the operation of the state extends. Furthermore, this primary human sociality, this primary need for others to need me and want me to abide in the world with them, expresses itself in adulthood when most of us choose to remain in the societies into which we were born or adopted and, indeed, to contribute to both the survival and the caring mission of our society. If humans discover that their society is not primarily devoted to the care of human beings, however, they have a moral obligation to either work for change in their society or leave it for another society. If humans discover that their society is primarily devoted to the destruction of human beings, they have a moral obligation to work for its utter defeat. (Consider, for example, anti-Nazi non-Jews in Germany in the 1930s, such as Pastor Dietrich Bonhoeffer, who realized they were powerless to change the murderous Nazi regime under which they were living and actively worked for its downfall.)

For a society's claims on any of its individual members to be accepted in good faith, each member of that society must feel himself or herself loyal to that society. All members of the society must be convinced that their welfare is the prime concern of that society. Many modern political theorists make the mistake of assuming that a direct relationship of mutual loyalty between a society and its members can be posited, and the familial relationship can be ignored or made tangential to the true social reality, which for them is the state. That view was first proposed by Plato, who projected an ideal society in which, at least for the governing class, individuals do not even know who their parents are and therefore cannot possibly have what anyone could cogently call a family.[116] For Plato, that arrangement seemed to be an improvement over the usual situation, in which a person's loyalty rarely extends to society as a whole.

As Aristotle soberly pointed out, however, persons who have not been socialized in the most immediate society possible—the family—do not bypass the part and simply transfer their loyalty directly to the whole. Instead, they have no loyalty to any human association at all.[117] Today, such people often become what we call sociopaths— that is, not only do they not have deep social ties; perhaps because of that lack of ties, they are inherently hostile to any society. We see this phenomenon especially among persons who, in the absence of families (whether that absence is total or because their families are grossly dysfunctional), have had to depend on the relatively impersonal welfare institutions of the state for their primary care. In these cases, the state can only do badly, for the most part, what more intimate families can do well, for the most part.

Following Aristotle's point against Plato, we could say that the effectiveness of a society that indicates to its members that it wants all of them to live and not die, by somebody else's hand or even by their own hand, largely depends on how much it respects the integrity of its families and respects and supports families' ability to care for their members in a way the state can supplement but not replace. The first message a family should send to all of its members, from the youngest to the oldest, is this: We want you to abide with us together in the world. There is no substitute for hearing that message from the people to whom one is tied through kinship. The task of the state in its overall welfare function is to assist families in sending that message to every person in their midst. Based on my past experience as a hospital chaplain and congregational rabbi, I think that very few persons who hear that kind message from their family (including a family into whom one is adopted, whether in childhood or adulthood) will want to die, let alone kill themselves and seek the help and approval of strangers in doing so. They do not want to abandon those for whom they care and who want to care for them.

Unfortunately, the persons who are nearest to us sometimes send the opposite message: We want you to die, so save us the trouble and the guilt and eliminate yourself for us. Alas, many people who hear that message heed its intent. For example, the suicide rate of German Jews increased dramatically after January 1933, with the nazification of Germany under Hitler—several years before the "Final Solution" with the death camps was implemented.[118] One might conclude that the explanation for this increase was that the society to which German Jews and their families looked for validation of their very existence in the world sent the brutally clear message that their presence must eliminate itself or be eliminated. Suicide offered the people who had been so rejected a gruesome option that many of them must have felt left them with at least some control over their own existence, however final.

The social needs of humans are coeval with their existence in the world. That existence itself is essentially to be with and for others and to have others be with and for us. The Talmud reports the cry of a sage who had been forgotten by the persons who were closest to him: "Either fellowship [*haveruta*] or death!"[119] In fact, that is the meaning of death. Death is not nonbeing, which is something no one has ever experienced or can even imagine. Instead, death is our own ultimate loneliness, our anticipation of being abandoned to our ultimate privacy. That is what death meant to Job, who in his misery felt himself to be dead already: "My kin have distanced themselves from me, and my friends are indeed estranged [*zaru*] from me; those who were close to me have ceased being close, and those who knew me have forgotten me" (Job 19: 13–14).[120] Because all of us have experienced loneliness, all of us can readily imagine what ultimate abandonment might be. That is why we all fear death and why most of us, most of the time, do everything we can to postpone its sting. Most of us could not do that, especially at times of great suffering and uncertainty, without the concern and the help of the others with whom and not just among whom we live. That is why some people who do not feel that they have such close familial-communal ties attempt to preempt death by becoming death itself and thus believing that they escape becoming death's passive victims. They take matters into their own hands because they want to actively abandon people they believe have already abandoned them.

Along these lines, we can learn much from the example of the Hutterites, a group of Christian pietists (somewhat similar to the Amish), most of whom live in remote regions of upper Canada and the upper Midwest of the United States. The Hutterites—who usually marry only other Hutterites, thus narrowing their gene pool—have a high instance of bipolar or manic-depressive illness in their community. (Many scientists now are of the opinion that there is a genetic predisposition to bipolar illness.) People with bipolar disorder have a high suicide rate, especially when they are in the depressive stage of their illness. Yet the Hutterites have an extremely low suicide rate. Why? It seems to be because when they notice the onset of the depression—which they call *Anfechtung* (literally, "an attack")—they never leave those persons suffering the depression alone.[121] They help these sufferers get through their depression alive by not abandoning them to their own self-caused death. That behavior is human and humane community in its greatest depth. One cannot imagine any Hutterite seeking any assistance from a physician who advocates his or her willingness to assist anybody in committing suicide.

STRUGGLING AGAINST THE POLITICS OF DEATH

There seems to be little likelihood that suicide will soon or ever again be designated a crime. Such a designation seems to most people to be blaming the victim, which is always the case when the criminal and the victim are the same person. Although we could regard criminalization of suicide ultimately as an effort to save lives and thus an instance of society's care for its distressed members, most people today would not see that connection; most would take such legislation to be cruel. Making the connection between the legal prohibition of suicide and the state as caregiver is simply too difficult, in terms of effective political argument or rhetoric. Probably the most that can be done on the legal front is to argue for penalization of anyone—especially physicians licensed by the state—who assists somebody else in committing suicide. The reason to be presented in this line of public argument should be that we regard all suicides to be the tragic result of mental illness (even if the persons committing suicide do not manifest the usual signs of clinical depression such as melancholia) and that no person should do anything to encourage, let alone facilitate, such an outcome.

We also should do everything we can to inform the public that physician-assisted suicide is not really an autonomous choice. More often than not, it could be regarded as the result of society sending a message through one of its officials—a licensed physician: We don't want you to be alive anymore because you are now useless to us and even to yourself; indeed, you will never be of any use to anyone ever again. Furthermore, there are powerful economic interests that would and probably do attempt to influence the state to send this message, such as insurance companies that insure the health care of most Americans (except for the more than 40 million Americans with no medical insurance). These companies would save huge amounts of money if the average lifespan of their clients were shorter, and they would not have to pay for extended end-of-life care. In this vision, physician-assisted suicide, in fact, increasingly becomes a pattern in which patients assist their physicians in killing them through "death with dignity" rather than the physicians carrying out the autonomous choice of their patients. If this pattern were to become the norm, many patients would have no autonomy any more because, based on the very prevalence of assisted suicide, society might decide that the average age at which most persons are likely to request suicide should be the age at which insurance benefits should end, even for the minority who do not want to die. Thus, even if society still recognizes our "autonomy"—our right to die or not die by our own choice—exercising one's right to continued medical treatment will be difficult if the institutions that pay for one's health care no longer will do so. Having only one real choice does not seem like freedom, let alone autonomy.

Finally, we should address the real concern of many people that they will have to die in agony, hooked up to machines, in a cold and impersonal institutional setting. That scenario has been presented to many people as their inevitable lot when they cannot end their own lives when they want to do so. Countering the moral conclusion drawn from the image of that scenario requires developing more effective treatments for pain relief and better informing the public of effective pain relief that is already available. We also should do more to enable more people to die in their own homes, surrounded by the people who love them, or in hospices dedicated to seeing that the patients for whom they care do not die by themselves.[122] Persons in these settings also are unlikely to be kept alive by "extraordinary means" for the sake of medical experimentation (even if physicians are keeping them alive only to gather data from their case)—something else many people fear. All of this rhetoric and political action depends on our ability to show the members of our own society that caring for one another—which minimally means protecting everybody from harm as much as possible—is the most attractive vision of even a secular society's *raison d'être*. We need to argue against the alternatives to that vision: a society whose *raison d'être* is the enhancement of its own power in the world or a society whose *raison d'être* is merely protection of its members' property. We need to argue that these visions of the main task of society are unworthy of human beings who are more than parts of an all-encompassing social whole and more than economic monads that are essentially alone in the world.

NOTES

The following abbreviations for classical Jewish sources are used throughout these notes:

B.   *Babylonian Talmud (Bavli)*

M.   *Mishnah*

MT   *Mishneh Torah* (Maimonides)

T.   *Tosefta*

Tos.   *Tosafot*

Y.   *Palestinian Talmud (Yerushalmi)*

Unless otherwise noted, all translations are by the author.

1. See D. Novak, *Law and Theology in Judaism*, vol. 1 (New York: KTAV, 1974), 83–86.
2. See Moses Schreiber, *Sheelot u-Teshuvot Hatam Sofer:* Yoreh Deah (Vienna: n.p., 1855), no. 326; B. Hullin 39b and Rashi, s.v. "im me'atsmo nafal"; Y. Sanhedrin 6.5/23c; see also Novak, *Law and Theology in Judaism*, vol. 1, 86–93.
3. See. B. Kiddushin 39b (opinion of R. Jacob).
4. See B. Makkot 10b; Maimonides, MT: Rotseah, 6.1–5.
5. See B. Sanhedrin 41a; see also David Novak, *The Jewish Social Contract* (Princeton, N.J.: Princeton University Press, 2005), 106.

6. Two of the most important articles dealing with this question are Timothy E. Quill et al., "Care of the Hopelessly Ill: Proposed Clinical Criteria for Physician-Assisted Suicide," *New England Journal of Medicine* 327 (1992): 1380–83; Franklin Miller and John Fletcher, "The Case for Legalized Euthanasia," *Perspectives in Biology and Medicine* 36 (1993): 159–76.

7. See Yale Kamisar, "The Reason So Many People Support Physician-Assisted Suicide—and Why These Reasons Are Not Convincing," *Issues in Law and Medicine* 12 (1996): 113–31; Daniel Callahan and Margot White, "The Legalization of Physician-Assisted Suicide: Creating a Potemkin Village," *University of Richmond Law Review* 30 (1996). 1–83.

8. See *Beresheet Rabbah* 34.13, ed. J. Theodor and C. Albeck (Jerusalem: Wahrmann, 1965), 324 and notes thereon.

9. See C. W. Reines, "The Jewish Attitude toward Suicide," *Judaism* 10 (1961): 170.

10. Only the death of a convicted criminal is "good for him and good for the world" (M. Sanhedrin 6.5). Yet even this person is entitled, minimally, to a decent burial. See T. Sanhedrin 9.11; B. Sanhedrin 46b; *cf.* ibid. 47a regarding Ps. 15:4.

11. See. B. Shabbat 151b.

12. See *Semahot* 2.1.

13. See B. Sanhedrin 39b regarding Ezek. 11:12.

14. B. Baba Kama 91b; Maimonides, MT: Hovel u-Maziq, 5.1 regarding Deut. 25:3; see also *Sifre: Devarim*, no. 286, and Y. Sanhedrin 11.1/30a regarding Deut. 25:3.

15. At most, a person making such a request has violated the proscription regarding "placing a stumbling-block before the blind" (Lev. 19:14), which means enticing someone else to sin—in this case the other person one has requested to perform one's own suicide. Because the request is only a verbal act, however, the one making this lethal request is not subject to any humanly administered punishment. See T. Makkot 5.10; B. Makkot 16a and parallels; Maimonides, MT: Sanhedrin, 18.1. See also II Sam. 1:9–10; B. Yevamot 78b; Novak, *Law and Theology in Judaism*, vol. 1, 90–93.

16. See *supra*, 47–50.

17. B. Kiddushin 43a. *Cf.* M. Berakhot 5.5. See *Beresheet Rabbah* 34.14 and R. Issachar Baer Katz, *Mattnot Kehunah* thereon (in *Midrash Rabbah* [New York: E. Grossman, 1957]).

18. B. Berakhot 9a and parallels.

19. It does seem, however, that Haggai is being cited as any other sage would be cited in the Talmud, not because of his extraordinary, prophetic authority. See B. Bekhorot 58a and Tos., s.v. "mi-pi Haggai." See also B. Baba Metsia 59b regarding Deut. 30:12.

20. B. Kiddushin 42b. See *Encyclopedia Talmudit*, vol. 1, 338–42.

21. See M. Baba Metsia 7.11 and parallels.

22. B. Kiddushin 42b.

23. Ibid. 43a.

24. Ibid. 42b and Rashi, s.v. "ein sheliah." The question of indirect causation of a forbidden act (*grama*) exempting the actor from legal liability in this world is complicated. See B. Baba Kama 56a and Tos., s.v. "ela"; ibid. 60a and Tos., s.v. "Rav Ashi." Even when there is *grama*, there is still moral guilt (*be-dinei shamayim*), whether there is any malicious intent or not. See Menahem ha-Meiri, *Bet ha-Behirah:* B. Baba Kama 56a, ed. K. Schlesinger (Jerusalem: n.p. 1967), 169–71.

25. *Commentary on the Earlier Prophets:* II Samuel, chap. 11.

26. II Sam. 1:14–24.

27. For Abravanel's low opinion of kingship in general because of the probability of the abuse of monarchial power, see his *Commentary on the Torah:* Deut. 17:14–20; see also Novak, *The Jewish Social Contract*, 150–56.

28. See B. Kiddushin 43a regarding II Sam. 11:11. When Maimonides discusses the illegitimate orders of King Ahab to kill Naboth the Jezreelite (I Kings 21:7–13), he speaks of Ahab as having "caused" [*seebev*] Naboth's death, but not by his own hand (MT: Sanhedrin, 4.9). In presenting the standard rabbinic interpretation of "you shall not place a stumbling-block before the blind" (Lev. 19:14 and *Sifra: Qedoshim*, ed. I. H. Weiss [Vienna: Schlessinger, 1862], 88d), meaning enabling someone else to sin, Maimonides speaks of the one who "causes" (*yesabev*) the sin to be actually committed by someone else. See *Sefer ha-Mitsvot:* neg. no. 299, Heb. trans. Ibn Tibbon, ed. C. Heller (Jerusalem: Mosad ha-Rav Kook, 1946), 172a. Hence the "cause" of the sin is the necessary (i.e., the person committing the sin couldn't have committed it without the "help" of this other person) but not sufficient cause of the forbidden act. The sole sufficient cause of the act is the person who was so enabled to do it and actually did it. He or she thus bears sole responsibility for the act itself. In fact, however, Maimonides more often uses the term *gorem* to describe such "enablers." See, e.g., *Commentary on the Mishnah:* Sheviit 5.6; ibid.: Terumot 6.3; MT: Genevah, 5.1. Furthermore, along these

lines, see M. Baba Metsia 5.11 and B. Baba Metsia 75b regarding Lev. 19:14.

29. See II Samuel 18:5–15, 29–32; 19:6–9.

30. The classic statement of this position is still that of John Stuart Mill, *On Liberty,* ed. G. Williams (London: J. M. Dent, 1993), 78–79.

31. B. Avodah Zarah 18a.

32. See, e.g., B. Berakhot 61b.

33. B. Avodah Zarah 18a.

34. Ibid. See *Semahot* 2.1 (statement of R. Ishmael).

35. See the commentary of the Tosafists, *Daat Zeqenim:* Gen. 9:5 (in *Miqraot Gedolot*).

36. *Cf.,* e.g., Abraham ibn Zimra, *Radbaz* on Maimonides, MT: Sanhedrin, 18.6 regarding Ezek. 18:4.

37. Deut. 20:19. See Maimonides, *Sefer ha-Mitsvot:* neg. no. 57.

38. Regarding the image of God as the basis of human inviolability, see *supra,* 24–25.

39. *Sifra:* Behar, 109c, and B. Baba Metsia 62a regarding Lev. 25:36; see also David Novak, *Covenantal Rights* (Princeton, N.J.: Princeton University Press, 2000), 122–31.

40. That is how the old English bibles translated *aphāken to pneuma* in Matthew 27:50 and *exepneusen* in Luke 23:46, speaking of the death of Jesus (also someone who was executed by the Romans as a revolutionary). These Greek terms no doubt are translations of the Hebrew *yetsi'at neshamah* and hence part of the lingua franca of first- and second-century CE Palestine. See M. Shabbat 23.5; B. Shabbat 151b.

41. See, e.g., Gen. 2:7; Ezek. 37:6; Eccl. 12:7. See also B. Berakhot 5a regarding Ps. 31:6.

42. Even criminals sentenced to death by a Jewish court were to be executed quickly and as painlessly as possible, as well as in a way that did not grossly disfigure the corpse. See B. Sanhedrin 43a regarding Prov. 31:6; ibid. 45a (and Rashi, s.v. "Meetah yafah" and "menuval"); ibid. 52a; Y. Sanhedrin 6.8/23c regarding Lev. 19:18; see also M. Halbertal, *Mehapehot Parshaniyot be-Hit'havutan* (Jerusalem: Magnes Press, 1997), 149–59. The tannaitic term *meetah yafah* may come from the Greek *euthuthanatos,* which means a "quick and easy death." See Plutarch, *Antony,* sec. 76, *Plutarch's Lives,* vol. 9, trans. B. Perrin (Cambridge, Mass.: Harvard University Press, 1959), 310–11. The modern term "euthanasia" might have been based on this classical source. The first modern use of this term I find is in the work of the classicist

W. E. H. Lecky, *History of Western Morals*, 3rd rev. ed. (New York: Appleton, 1898), vol. 1, 221. (The first edition of this famous work was published in 1869). To be sure, the term *euthanasia* does appear in Hellenistic sources (see, e.g., Philo, *De Sacrificiis*, 100), which themselves drew on earlier Greek sources, both dramatic and philosophic (see, e.g., Sophocles, *Oedipus Rex*, 1929–30; Aristotle, *Nicomachean Ethics*, 1.10/1100a10-15). In these sources, however, *euthanasia*, which literally means "good dying," seems to refer to a natural process (like *eugeria*, meaning "good old age") rather than a humanly caused event such as *euthusthanatos*, which literally means "a quick death." Whereas one can know whether one will have *euthusthanatos* because it is an act that is intended *ab initio*, one can know whether one has had *euthanasia* only after one has died; that is, it can be known only *post factum*.

43. Later sources, however, permit one to pray that God take one's own life or the life of somebody else when that body is suffering excruciating, interminable pain. See I Kings 19:4–15; Jonah 4:3–11; B. Ketubot 39b–40a and Nissim Gerondi (Ran), s.v. "ein mevaqesh" thereon. See also see B. Yoma 83a regarding Prov. 14:10 for the notion that a person himself or herself knows how much pain he or she can stand. *Cf.* B. Ketubot 33b.

44. See E. L. Fackenheim, *To Mend the World* (New York: Schocken, 1982), 201–25.

45. See B. Baba Kama 28b regarding Deut. 22:26; B. Yevamot 55b–56a and Tos., s.v. "ein ones"; Maimonides, MT: Yesodei ha-Torah, 5.4.

46. *Sifra:* Qedoshim, 88d.

47. Maimonides, *Commentary on the Mishnah:* Terumot 6.3, Heb. trans. Y. Kafih, 183.

48. See B. Avodah Zarah 55a; Maimonides, *Commentary on the Mishnah:* Sheviit 5.6; MT: Rotseah, 12.14 regarding B. Avodah Zarah 15b.

49. See T. Makkot 5.10; B. Makkot 16a; B. Sanhedrin 63a–b and parallels; Maimonides, MT: Gezelah, 5.1.

50. See also *Midrash Leqah Tov:* Lev. 19:14.

51. See also *Zohar* 3: Vayiqra, 85a.

52. MT: Malveh ve-Loveh, 4.2 regarding B. Baba Metsia 75b (see Tos., s.v. "arav" thereon).

53. B. Avodah Zarah 6a–b: Rabbenu Hananeal, Rashi (s.v. "de-qayyama"), and Tos., s.v. "minayyin" thereon.

54. *Sifra:* Qedoshim, 88d.

55. There are two kinds of "fear of God" (*yir'at ha-shem*): being in awe of God as the Creator of all being and being afraid of what God can do

to oneself. For this differentiation, see *Zohar* 1: intro., 11b. The first kind of *yir'ah* is termed "essential" (*iqqara*); the second is termed "nonessential" (*l'av iqqara*)—that is, secondary.

56. If and what a patient is to be told about his or her condition depends on the assessment of his or her caretakers regarding whether the patient can rationally deal with such information or not. See Nahmanides, *Torat ha'Adam:* Inyan ha-Vidui, 46; *Tur* and *Shulhan Arukh: Yoreh Deah*, 338.1.

57. Along these lines, one need only fulfill the commandment "you shall surely warn [*hokehah tokheah*] your neighbor" (Lev. 19:17) when one can be reasonably sure that the person to be warned will properly heed the warning. See B. Yevamot 65b regarding Prov. 9:8.

58. See B. Yoma 83a regarding Prov. 14:10, and David Halivni, *Meqorot u-Mesorot:* Moed (Jerusalem: Jewish Theological Seminary of America, 1975) thereon, 141–42.

59. In Jewish law, the principle of double effect is used in the laws pertaining to violation of the Sabbath. Because connections have been made between the laws pertaining to human life and the laws pertaining to the Sabbath (see, e.g., B. Yoma 85b regarding Exod. 31:14), we may be able to use the principle of double effect as developed in Sabbath law to deal with double effect in the issue of physician-assisted suicide. With regard to violation of the Sabbath, one is not guilty (*patur*) when one intended to do something permitted, and the prohibited act happened to occur along with it—accidentally, as it were. One would be liable (*hayyav*), however, if the secondary act was intended (*mitkavven*); the secondary act occurred inevitably along with the primary, permitted act; and the secondary act produced some definite, desirable, and tangible benefit for that person, even if it was not intended *ab initio*. See B. Shabbat 41b; ibid. 75a and Tos., s.v. "tfei neeha leih."

60. See Menahem ha-Meiri, *Bet ha-Behirah:* B. Baba Kama 56a regarding Ps. 44:22, 171.

61. *Sefer ha-Mitsvot:* neg. no. 289, 172.

62. B. Berakhot 32b–33a.

63. Ibid. 32b. See Maimonides, MT: Tefillah, 6.9. One is to die as a martyr only if one is forced to commit idolatry, sexual license, or murder. See B. Sanhedrin 75a–b; Maimonides, MT: Yesodei ha-Torah, 5.1-10.

64. B. Shevuot 36a; B. Eruvin 96a and parallels.

65. For a profound philosophical discussion of this whole problem, see Paul Riceour, *Oneself as Another,* trans. K. Blamey (Chicago: University of Chicago Press, 1992), 319–29.

66. See *Mekhilta:* Mishpatim, 327; M. M. Kasher, *Torah Shlemah:* Exod. 23:7, n. 107.

67. There is considerable halakhic opinion that one is not considered to have been a willful suicide unless one was forewarned (*hatra'ah*) by someone else and explicitly rejected this forewarning. See Jacob Weill, *Sheelot u-Teshuvot Mahari Weill,* no. 114; Moses Isserles, *Darkhei Mosheh* on *Tur:* Yoreh Deah, sec. 345, n. 3; Y. Y. Greenwald, *Kol Bo al Avelut,* 4.3 (New York: Feldheim, 1965), 320. Therefore, one might say that anyone who does not attempt to talk a would-be suicide out of committing suicide when confronted by such a person, by whatever means are judged appropriate for that would-be suicide, is guilty of violating the prohibition "you shall not stand idly by the blood of your neighbor" (Lev. 19:16). See B. Sanhedrin 73a and esp. Maimonides, MT: Rotseah, 1.14 (which could easily be extended to include saving somebody from himself or herself).

68. M. Baba Kama 8.6.

69. B. Baba Kama 91b.

70. See B. Berakhot 34b regarding Isa. 64:3.

71. See Maimonides, MT: Teshuvah, 2.1–2.

72. See Abraham ibn Ezra, *Commentary on the Torah:* Gen. 9:5.

73. See *Beresheet Rabbah* 34.13–14.

74. See Israel Lifschuetz, *Tiferet Yisrael* on M. Sanhedrin 10.2; see also A. Perls, "Der Selbstmord nach der Halacha," *Monatschrift für die Geschichte und Wissenschaft des Judenthums* 55 (1911), 288, n. 6.

75. See Epictetus, *Discourses,* 1.24; Seneca, *Epistolae,* 70. "Ecstasy" comes from the Greek *ek histēmi,* meaning "to stand outside [of oneself]." *Cf.* B. Berakhot 10a regarding *neshamah* taken to be a separate substance like "soul" (*psychē*) for Plato and earlier Greek thinkers and the Stoics who largely followed him. See David Novak, *Suicide and Morality* (New York: Scholars Studies Press, 1975), 8–19.

76. See *Encyclopedia Miqraeet,* 5:898–900, s.v. "nefesh."

77. See M. Sanhedrin 10.1; B. Taanit 2a–b regarding Ezek. 37:13.

78. Reinhold Niebuhr, *The Nature and Destiny of Man,* vol. 2 (New York: Chas. Scribner's Sons, 1943), 311–12.

79. See, e.g., Ps. 49:13–21; Eccl. 3:19–20.

80. Plato, *Republic,* 431A, trans. P. Shorey (Cambridge, Mass.: Harvard University Press, 1930), vol. 1, 358–59. See Aristotle, *Nicomachean Ethics,* 5.11/1138b6–11.

81. See Plato, *Euthyphro,* 10A–E.

82. See *Republic,* 523A–525A.

83. At times, such reliance on greater expertise is appropriate, as long as experience has taught us that such expertise deserves its authority because of its regular conformity with the law of God. See M. Horayot 1.1; B. Horayot 2a; Y. Horayot 1.1/45c regarding Lev. 4:1 and ibid. 45d regarding Deut. 17:11. Clearly, a suicide-prescribing physician is not in that category.

84. For an insightful discussion of the difference between freedom of choice (*liberum arbitrium*) and freedom of the will (*Willensfreiheit*), see Hannah Arendt, *The Life of the Mind*, vol. 2: Willing (New York and London: Harcourt Brace Jovanovich, 1978), 26–34, 84–110.

85. See B. Baba Batra 10b regarding Prov. 21:24.

86. See B. Sotah 14a regarding Deut. 13:5; Maimonides, *Guide of the Perplexed*, 3.54 regarding Jer. 9:23.

87. See *Sifre: Devarim*, no. 329 regarding Deut. 22:8; B. Shabbat 32a. Regarding the assumption that everything that happens to us is from God's will, see B. Hullin 7b regarding Ps. 37:23 and Prov. 20:24. Nevertheless, that does not mean that everything done by us was willed by God for us to do because that would deny our freedom of choice and its attendant responsibility. See B. Berakhot 33b regarding Deut. 10:12; Maimonides, MT: Teshuvah, chaps. 5–6. We need to take more responsibility for the evil we do than for the good we do because we do evil on the basis of our sense of our own autonomy, but when we do good properly, we do so for the sake of God and on God's behalf.

88. See B. Sanhedrin 6b regarding II Sam. 8:15 (interpretation of Rebbi); see also M. Makkot 3.15 and Maimonides, *Commentary on the Mishnah* thereon; B. Makkot 13b and Rashi, s.v. "Rabbi Akiva."

89. Gen. 3:12–14.

90. MT: Sanhedrin, 18.6.

91. See, e.g., Lev. 5:20–26, and *Sifra: Vayiqra*, 27d.

92. M. Sanhedrin 6.2 regarding Josh. 7:19–25.

93. Ibid. See B. Eruvin 19a regarding Ps. 65:2.

94. See Aristotle, *Nicomachean Ethics*, 6.1-5/1139a5–1141a9.

95. See David Novak, *Natural Law in Judaism* (Cambridge: Cambridge University Press, 1998), chap. 1.

96. Brandeis presented that phrase in an article he co-authored more than twenty-five years before his appointment as an associate justice of the U.S. Supreme Court. See Samuel D. Warren and Louis D. Brandeis, "The Right to Privacy," *Harvard Law Review* 4 (1890): 193. That article has had enormous influence on contemporary jurisprudence.

For a critique of that line of thinking, however, see David Novak, *Covenantal Rights* (Princeton, N.J.: Princeton University Press, 2000), 2–25.

97. For an application of this notion to the issue of physician-assisted suicide, see John Linville, "Physician-Assisted Suicide as a Constitutional Right," *Journal of Law, Medicine, and Ethics* 24 (1996): 198–206.

98. Immanuel Kant, *Groundwork of the Metaphysic of Morals*, trans. H. J. Paton (New York: Harper and Row, 1964), 80–102. Even Locke, who seems to have a more individualistic ethics than that of Kant, nonetheless regards natural sociality and its inherent restraints as operating within the "state of nature," even before persons have to enter civil society with its new, invented, political restraints. See John Locke, *Second Treatise of Civil Government*, chap. 2.

99. See the decision of U.S. Court of Appeals Judge Stephen Reinhardt in *Compassion in Dying v. Washington*, 79F.3d 790 (1996).

100. See Aristotle, *Nicomachean Ethics*, 5.2/1130b30–1131a9.

101. See *supra*, chap. 2.

102. Aristotle, *Nicomachean Ethics*, 5.11/1138b6.

103. Ibid., 5.11/1138a9–15, rev. ed., trans. H. Rackham (Cambridge, Mass.: Harvard University Press, 1934), 318–19. Aristotle speaks of one "who kills himself in a fit of passion" (*di'orgēn*). Although "voluntary," such an angry act is not deliberately chosen. Yet that person is responsible for his angry act of self-destruction because, even though he did not intend to kill himself, he still could have prevented the suicide by not giving in to his anger *ab initio*, the passion that blindly led him to end his own life. See ibid., 3.1/1109b30–1110a15. The question Aristotle does not address, however, is against whom this anger is directed.

104. See Aristotle, *Politics*, 1.1/1252b29–1253a5.

105. Ibid., 8.1/1337a26–30.

106. Interestingly enough, Plato, whose ethical teaching was more theologically inclined than that of Aristotle, is closer to the Jewish tradition when he states that suicide deprives God of what is His. See *Phaedo*, 62C. *Cf.* Ezek. 18:4. Moreover, one could ask whether Aristotle would have agreed with Plato (see *Crito*, 50A–52A) that a citizen has the right to leave a *polis* such as Athens by emigrating—before one has committed a crime for which one is obligated to accept one's punishment from the *polis*, as Socrates did. Yet one could say that suicide is different inasmuch as it is not a crime of abandonment of the *polis* but a crime of hostility, in the form of robbery, that is committed

against the *polis.* That is not the case, however, when one emigrates *from* the *polis* to settle somewhere else. Hence, Plato's condemnation of suicide in *Laws,* 873C–D does not contradict *Crito,* 50A–52A.

107. See Novak, *Suicide and Morality,* 59–64.

108. Plato, *Laws,* 873C–D, vol. 1, trans. R. G. Bury (Cambridge, Mass.: Harvard University Press, 1926), 264–65.

109. See Plato, *Apology,* 24B–C; *Phaedo,* 57A.

110. See Plato, *Phaedo,* 117C. Of course, Socrates would do this only because it was a commandment of a god. Hence, he consistently refused to kill himself as an autonomous act (see *Crito,* 54E; *Phaedo,* 62A only D). Killing himself would have been, for Socrates, as impious as running away from Athens as a criminal fugitive and thereby showing his contempt for Athenian law, which had divine or holy status for him (see *Crito,* 51B). Along these lines, could we not say that one who commits suicide as the dutiful response to the claim made upon one by an official of the state, such as a state-licensed physician, is thereby ascribing divine or semi-divine status to that physician (as Socrates ascribed to Athenian law and its officials) because of one's unquestioned acceptance of a prescription that physician made?

111. This position goes far beyond what Locke (whom many liberals often cite as precedent) thought. For Locke, we own the labor of our bodies and what this labor produces. Our right to that labor is given to us, along with the earth—which is given to humans to use for their benefit. We do not own our bodies per se, however. Ownership of our bodies belongs to God. Thus, Locke works out his theory of property from a theology of creation. See John Locke, *Second Treatise of Civil Government,* ed. G. B. McPherson (Indianapolis: Hackett, 1980), 5.27, 44. Indeed, at the very beginning of this section of the treatise on property, Locke quotes Ps. 115:6 about how God "has given the earth to the children of men"—the earth, but not their own bodies.

112. See David Novak, "Can Capital Punishment Ever Be Justified in the Jewish Tradition?" in *Religion and the Death Penalty,* ed. E. C. Owens, J. D. Carlson, and E. P. Elshtain (Grand Rapids, Mich.: Eerdmans Publishing Co., 204), 31–47.

113. There is an interesting example in Jewish law of how one can be forced to do something in one's own best interest as an otherwise law-abiding member of society, especially when not doing this act will harm another member of this society. The case involves a man who refuses to divorce his wife when she has a right to such a divorce (*get*) from him, and he has been ordered by the court to give it to her.

Without this divorce, this woman is harmed because she cannot remarry until she obtains it. Because the husband must give the divorce to his wife willingly, the court forces him to do so as if it were his own will. Maimonides considers his recalcitrance to caused by what we might call temporary insanity. By forcing the man to give this divorce to his estranged wife, we are not only benefiting her, we also are benefiting her former husband by making him become once again a law-abiding, reputable member of society. See Maimonides, MT: Gerushin, 2.20 regarding M. Arakhin 5.6 (regarding Lev. 1:3); Novak, *Law and Theology in Judaism*, vol. 1, chap. 4. Such coercion, however, can only be the act of a duly constituted court as an official state institution, in a state governed by a just system of law that is attempting to prevent a great injustice from being done in its midst. See M. Gittin 9.8; B. Gittin 88b regarding Exod. 21:1 (second opinion). Accordingly, as in all proper incursions by the state into what is normally the realm of private individuals, this incursion is not for the sake of effecting the power of the state but to prevent an injustice being done by one individual to another or the common good of society. See B. Yevamot 89b re Ezra 10:8 and Tos., s.v. "keivan"; B. Baba Batra 99b–100a; Novak, *Covenantal Rights*, 209–13. When we prevent a suicide, are we not saving that person from himself or herself, and saving him or her for others as well?

114. See Plato, *Crito*, 51D–E.

115. See Aristotle, *Politics*, 1.1/1252b15–29.

116. Plato, *Republic*, 457D–461E.

117. Aristotle, *Politics*, 2.1/1261a5–1262b35. Importantly enough, in his more conservative political theory, Plato affirms the indispensable role of the family in a truly just society. See Plato, *Laws*, 689E–690A, 717B–718B, 869B–C.

118. See Saul Friedländer, *Nazi Germany and the Jews*, vol. 1 (New York: Harper Collins, 1997), 239–40, 276, 305.

119. B. Tanit 23a. See *Mahzor Vitry* on M. Avot 2.11, ed. S. Horovitz (Berlin: Z. H. Itzkovski, n.d.), 502.

120. Recall that Job's wife had urged him to commit suicide, telling him, "Curse God and die!" (Job 2:9). She no doubt thought God would strike Job dead on the spot for his blasphemy, or that blasphemy was a capital crime in their society and Job would be executed for it. Either way, the inevitable result would be the same as if he had taken his own life by his own hand. Job's wife seemed to be urging Job to get even with God who, for all intents and purposes, has killed Job already.

121. See John Hostetler, *Hutterite Society* (Baltimore and London: Johns Hopkins University Press, 1974), 262–68.

122. In the Jewish tradition, one is not to be left alone or with strangers at the time of one's death, if at all possible. See Joseph Karo, *Bet Yosef* on *Tur:* Yoreh Deah, 339; *Shulhan Arukh:* Yoreh Deah, 339.4 and note thereon regarding Ps. 49:10–11.

BIBLIOGRAPHY

CLASSICAL JUDAIC TEXTS

Abraham ibn Zimra (Radbaz). In Maimonides, *Mishneh Torah*.

Abravanel, Isaac. *Commentary on the Former Prophets*. Reprint. Jerusalem: Torah ve-Daat, 1956.

————. *Commentary on the Torah*. Warsaw: Lebensohn, 1862.

Albo, Joseph. *The Book of First Principles*. Edited and translated by I. Husik. 5 vols. Philadelphia: Jewish Publication Society of America, 1929–1930.

Alfasi, Isaac (Rif). *Digest of the Talmud*. In *Babylonian Talmud*.

Arbaah Turim (Tur). 7 vols. Jerusalem: Feldheim, 1969.

Ashkenazi, Zvi. *Sheelot u-Teshuvot Hakham Zvi*. Amsterdam: n.p., 1712.

Babylonian Talmud (*Bavli*). 20 vols. Vilna: Romm, 1898.

Bachrach, Hayyim Yair. *Sheelot u-Teshuvot Havot Yair*. Reprint. Jerusalem: n.p., 1973.

Bemidbar Rabbah. In *Midrash Rabbah*.

Beresheet Rabbah. Edited by J. Theodor and C. Albeck. 3 vols. Reprint. Jerusalem: Wahrmann, 1965.

Chajes, Zvi Hirsch. *Hagahot ve-Hiddushim*. In *Babylonian Talmud*, Vilna ed.

————. *Kol Kitvei Maharats Chajes*. 2 vols. Jerusalem: Divrei Hakhamim, 1958.

Daat Zeqenim. In *Miqraot Gedolot: Pentateuch*.

Elijah Gaon of Vilna (Gra). *Commentary on the Latter Prophets*. Jerusalem: Feldheim, n.d.

Halakhot Gedolot. 2 vols. Edited by E. Hildesheimer. Reprint. Jerusalem: Mekitse Nirdamim, 1971.

Hananeal (Rabbenu). In *Babylonian Talmud*, Vilna ed.

Ibn Ezra, Abraham. *Commentary on the Torah*. 3 vols. Edited by A. Weiser. Jerusalem: Mosad ha-Rav Kook, 1977.

Isserles, Moses. *Darkhe Mosheh*. In *Arbaah Turim*.

————. *Hagahot*. In: *Shulhan Arukh*.

Karo, Joseph. *Bet Yosef*. In *Tur*.

Katz, Issachar Baer. *Mattnot Ketunah*. In *Midrash Rabbah*.

Kesef Mishneh. In Maimonides, *Mishneh Torah*.

————. *Shulhan Arukh.* 7 vols. Lemberg: n.p., 1873.

Landau, Ezekiel. *Sheelot u-Teshuvot Noda Bi-Yehudah.* Reprint. Jerusalem: n.p., 1960. Lieberman, Saul. *Tosefta Kifshuta.* 12 vols. New York: Jewish Theological Seminary of America, 1955–1988.

Lifschuetz, Israel. *Tiferet Yisrael.* In *Mishnayot.* 12 vols. Reprint. New York: M. P. Press, 1969.

Luria, David. *Hiddushei Radal.* In *Midrash Rabbah.*

Mahzor Vitry. Edited by S. Hurwitz. Berlin: Z. H. Itzkovski, n.d.

Maimonides, Moses. *Commentary on the Mishnah.* Translated by Y. Kafih. 3 vols. Jerusalem: Mosad ha-Rav Kook, 1964–1967.

————. *Guide of the Perplexed.* Translated by S. Pines. Chicago: University of Chicago Press, 1963.

————. *Mishneh Torah.* 5 vols. Reprint. New York: E. Grossman, 1957.

————. *Sefer ha-Mitsvot.* Edited by C. Heller. Jerusalem: Mosad ha-Rav Kook, 1946.

————. *Shemonah Peraqim.* In *Commentary on the Mishnah.*

Margolies, Mosheh. *Pnei Mosheh.* In *Palestinian Talmud,* Pietrkov ed.

Meir Abulafia. *Yad Ramah:* Sanhedrin. New York: Sifrei Qodesh, 1971.

Meir Simhah of Dvinsk. *Meshekh Hokhmah.* 3 vols. Edited by Y. Copperman. Jerusalem: Jerusalem College for Women, n.d.

Mekhilta de-Rabbi Ishmael. Edited by H. S. Horovitz and I. A. Rabin. Reprint. Jerusalem: Wahrmann, 1960.

Menachem ha-Meiri. *Bet ha-Behirah:* Baba Kamma. 3rd ed. Edited by K. Schlesinger. Jerusalem: n.p., 1967.

————. *Bet ha-Behirah:* Baba Batra. Edited by B. Menat. Jerusalem: n.p., 1971.

Midrash Leqah Tov. 2 vols. Edited by S. Buber. Vilna, 1884.

Midrash Rabbah. 2 vols. Reprint. New York: E. Grossman, 1957.

Miqraot Gedolot: Pentateuch. 5 vols. Reprint. New York: n.p., 1953.

Mishnah. 6 vols. Edited by C. Albeck. Tel Aviv: Mosad Bialik and Dvir, 1957.

Nahmanides, Moses. *Commentary on the Torah.* Edited by C. B. Chavel. 2 vols. Jerusalem: Mosad ha-Rav Kook, 1959–1963.

————. *Kitvei Ramban.* Edited by C. B. Chavel. 2 vols. Jerusalem: Mosad ha-Rav Kook, 1963.

————. *Torat ha-Adam.* In *Kitvei Ramban,* vol. 2.

Nissim Gerondi (Ran). Commentary on Alfasi (Rif). In Babylonian Talmud, Vilna ed.

Palestinian Talmud (*Yerushalmi*). Pietrkov ed. 7 vols. Reprint. Jerusalem: n.p., 1959.

————. Venice/Krotoschin ed. Reprint. New York: Yam ha-Talmud, 1948.

Radbaz. In *Mishneh Torah*.

Rashi. *Commentary* on Babylonian Talmud.

———. *Commentary on the Torah*. Edited by C. Chavel. Jerusalem: Mosad ha-Rav Kook, 1982.

Saadiah Gaon. *Book of Beliefs and Opinions*. Translated by S. Rosenblatt. New Haven, Conn.: Yale University Press, 1948.

Schreiber, Moses. *Teshuvot Hatam Sofer*. 5 vols. Vienna: n.p., 1855.

Sefer Hasidim. Bologna edition. Reprint. Jerusalem, 1966.

Semahot (Tractate: *Mourning*). Edited and translated by Dov Zlotnik. New Haven, Conn.: Yale University Press, 1966.

Septuagint. Edited by A. Rahlfs. 2 vols. Stuttgart: Privileg. Wurtt. Bibelanstalt, n.d.

Sifra. Edited by I. H. Weiss. Vienna: Schlessinger, 1862.

Sifre: Devarim. Edited by Louis Finkelstein. New York: Jewish Theological Seminary of America, 1969.

Sirachides (Ben Sira). In *Septuagint*.

Tanhuma. 2 vols. Edited by S. Buber. Reprint. Jerusalem: n.p., 1964.

Targum Jonathan ben Uzziel. In *Miqraot Gedolot:* Pentateuch, Prophets, and Writings.

Tosafot. In *Babylonian Talmud*, Vilna ed.

Tosefta. Edited by S. Zuckermandl. Reprint. Jerusalem: Wahrmann, 1937.

Tosefta: Zeraqim-Niziqin. 5 vols. Edited by Saul Lieberman. New York: Jewish Theological Seminary, 1955–1988.

Tur. See *Arbaah Turim*. 4 vols. Edited by M. Margoliot. Jerusalem: American Academy of Jewish Research, 1953–1956.

Vayiqra Rabbah. 4 vols. Edited by M. Margoliot. Jerusalem: American Academy of Jewish Research, 1953–1956.

Vidal of Tolosa. *Maggid Mishneh*. In Maimonides, *Mishneh Torah*.

Waldenberg, Eliezer. *Tsits Eliezer*. 2nd ed. Jerusalem: n.p., 1985.

Weill, Jacob. *Sheelot u-Teshuvot Mahari Weill*. Jerusalem: Tiferet haTorah, 1988.

Yom Tov ben Abraham Ishbili. *Hiddushei ha-Ritva*. 3 vols. Warsaw: n.p., 1902.

Zohar. Edited by R. Margaliot. 3 vols. Jerusalem: Mosad ha-Rav Kook, 1984.

MODERN JUDAIC TEXTS

Bleich, J. David. "In Vitro Fertilization: Questions of Maternal Identity and Conversion." *Tradition* 25, no. 4 (1991): 82–102.

Cohen, Hermann. *Jüdische Schriften*. 3 vols. Edited by B. Strauss. Berlin: C. A. Schwetschke, 1924.

————. *Religion of Reason Out of the Sources of Judaism*. Translated by S. Kaplan. New York: Frederick Unger, 1972.

Dorff, Elliot. *Matters of Life and Death*. Philadelphia: Jewish Publication Society, 1998.

Encyclopedia Miqareet. Jerusalem: Bialik Institute, 1982.

Encyclopedia Talmudit. 21 vols. Jerusalem, 1955–1963.

Fackenheim, Emil. *To Mend the World: Foundations of Future Jewish Thought*. New York: Schocken Books, 1982.

Feldman, D. M. *Birth Control in Jewish Law*. New York: New York University Press, 1968.

Ginzberg, Louis. *Legends of the Jews*. 7 vols. Philadelphia: Jewish Publication Society, 1909–1938.

Greenwald, Yekutiel Y. *Kol Bo al Avelut*. New York: Feldheim, 1965.

Halbertal, M. *Mehapehot Parshaniyot be-Hithavutan*. Jerusalem: Magnes Press, 1997.

Halivni, David Weiss. *Meqorot u-Masorot:* Nashim. Tel Aviv: Devir, 1968.

————. *Meqorot u-Masorot:* Moed. Tel Aviv: Devir, 1975.

Heschel, Abraham Joshua. *God in Search of Man*. New York: Farrar, Straus & Cudahy, 1955.

Jakobovits, Immanuel. *Jewish Medical Ethics: A Comparative and Historical Study of the Jewish Religious Attitude to Medicine and Its Practice*. New ed. New York: Bloch Publishing Co., 1975.

Kasher, Menachem. *Torah Shelemah*. 11 vols. Reprint. Jerusalem: M. M. Kasher, 1992.

Lichtenstein, Aharon. "Does the Jewish Tradition Recognize an Ethic Independent of Halakha?" In *Modern Jewish Ethics*, edited by M. Fox. Columbus: Ohio State University Press, 1975.

Novak, David. *Covenantal Rights*. Princeton, N.J.: Princeton University Press, 2000.

————. *The Election of Israel*. Cambridge: Cambridge University Press, 1995.

————. *Halakhah in a Theological Dimension*. Chico, Calif.: Scholars Press, 1985.

————. *The Image of the Non-Jew in Judaism*. New York: Edwin Mellen Press, 1983.

————. *The Jewish Social Contract*. Princeton, N.J.: Princeton University Press, 2005.

————. *Jewish Social Ethics*. New York: Oxford University Press, 1992.

————. *Law and Theology in Judaism*. 2 vols. New York: KTAV, 1974–1976.

————. *Natural Law in Judaism*. Cambridge: Cambridge University Press, 1998.

——. *Talking with Christians.* Grand Rapids, Mich.: Eerdmans Publishing Co., 2005.

——. *The Theology of Nahmanides Systemically Presented.* Atlanta: Scholars Press, 1992.

——. "Can Capital Punishment Ever Be Justified in the Jewish Tradition?" In *Religion and the Death Penalty,* edited by E. C. Owens, J. D. Carlson, and E. P. Elshtain. Grand Rapids, Mich.: Eerdmans Publishing Co., 2004: 31–47.

Perls, A. "Der Selbtsmord nach der Halacha." *Monatschrift für die Geschichte und Wissenschaft des Judenthums* 55 (1910): 287–95.

Reines, Chaim. "The Jewish Attitude toward Suicide." *Judaism* 10 (1961): 160–70.

Schiff, Daniel. *Abortion in Jewish Law.* Cambridge: Cambridge University Press, 2002.

Tendler, Moshe. "Rabbinic Comment: In Vitro Fertilization and Extrauterine Pregnancy." *Mount Sinai Journal of Medicine* 51 (1984): 7–11.

Tomeikh haHalakhah: Responsa of the Panel of Halakhic Inquiry. Edited by Wayne Allen. Teaneck, N.J.: Union for Traditional Judaism, 1994.

DENOMINATIONAL RESPONSES TO STEM CELL RESEARCH
Rabbinical Council of America: www.rabbis.org/news/article.cfm?id= 100553

United Synagogue of Conservative Judaism: www.uscj.org/Stem_Cell_Research_a6675.html

Union for Reform Judaism: http://urj.us/cgi-bin/resodisp.pl?file=stemcell &year=2003N

See also www.georgetown.edu/research/nrcbl/nbac/stemcell3.pdf

GENERAL TEXTS
Arendt, Hannah. *The Life of the Mind.* 2 vols. New York: Harcourt Brace Jovanovich, 1978.

Aristotle. *History of Animals.* Books 7–11. Translated by D. M. Balme. Cambridge, Mass.: Harvard University Press, 1991.

——. *Nicomachean Ethics.* Translated by H. Rackham. Cambridge, Mass.: Harvard University Press, 1926.

——. *Politics.* Translated by H. Rackham. Cambridge, Mass.: Harvard University Press, 1932.

Bible. Authorized King James Version. Oxford: Oxford University Press, 1998.

Brody, Baruch. *Abortion and the Sanctity of Human Life.* Cambridge, Mass.: MIT Press, 1975.

Buber, Martin. *Ich und Du*. Frankfurt am-Main: Insel-Verlag, 1923.

———. *I and Thou*. Translated by R. G. Smith. Edinburgh: T. and T. Clark, 1937.

———. *I and Thou*. Translated by W. Kaufmann. New York: Scribner's, 1970.

Callahan, Daniel, and Margot White. "The Legalization of Physician Assisted Suicide: Creating a Potemkin Village." *University of Richmond Law Review* 30 (1996): 1–83.

Carlson, Bruce. *Patten's Foundations of Embryology*. New York: McGraw Hill, 1996.

Condic, Maureen. "Stem Cells and Babies." *First Things* 155 (2005): 12–13.

Daar, A. S., and Lorraine Sheremata. "The Science of Stem Cells: Some Implications for Law and Policy." *Health Law Review* 11, no. 1 (2002): 5–13.

Dennis, Carina. "Cloning: Mining the Secrets of the Egg." *Nature* 439 (9 February 2006): 652–55.

Digest (Corpus Juris Civilis). In Bruce Freir, *A Casebook on the Roman Law of Delict*. Atlanta: Scholars Press, 1998.

Eliot, T. S. *Murder in the Cathedral*. In *The Complete Poems and Plays*. New York: Harcourt, Brace, and World, 1971.

Epictetus. *Discourses*. 2 vols. Translated by W. A. Oldfather. London: W. Heinemann, 1925–1928.

Freedman, Benjamin. *Duty and Healing*. New York and London: Routledge, 1999.

Friedländer, Saul. *Nazi Germany and the Jews*. Vol. 1. New York: Harper Collins, 1997.

Frier, Bruce. *A Casebook on the Roman Law of Delict*. Atlanta: Scholars Press, 1998.

Grisez, Germain. "The First Principle of Practical Reason: A Commentary on the *Summa Theologiae* 94.2." *Natural Law Forum* 10 (1965): 168–201.

Halevi, Haim David. "Fetal Reduction" (in Hebrew). *Assia* nos. 47–48 (12:3–4) (1990): 12–13.

Hegel, G. W. F. *Phänomenologie des Geistes*. Edited by J. Hoffmeister. Hamburg: Felix Meiner Verlag, 1952.

Hostetler, John. *Hutterite Society*. Baltimore and London: Johns Hopkins University Press, 1974.

Hume, David. *A Treatise of Human Nature*. Edited by L. A. Selby-Bigge. Oxford: Clarendon Press, 1888.

Jaspers, Karl. *Philosophy*. 3 vols. Translated by E. B. Ashton. Chicago and London: University of Chicago Press, 1969–1971.

Kant, Immanuel. *Critique of Practical Reason.* Translated by W. S. Pluhar. Indianapolis: Hackett, 2002.

————. *Critique of Pure Reason.* Translated by N. Kemp Smith. New York: St. Martin's Press, 1929.

————. *Groundwork of the Metaphysics of Morals.* Translated by H. J. Paton. New York: Harper and Row, 1964.

Kasimar, Yale. "The Reason So Many People Support Physician-Assisted Suicide—and Why These Reasons Are Not Convincing." *Issues in Law and Medicine* 12 (1996): 113–31.

Lecky, W. E. H. *History of European Morals.* 3rd rev. ed. 2 vols. New York: Appleton, 1898.

Levinas, Emmanuel. *Totality and Infinity.* Translated by A. Lingis. Pittsburgh: Duquesne University Press, 1969.

Liddell, H. G., and Scott, R. *A Greek-English Lexicon.* Rev. ed. Oxford: Clarendon Press, 1996.

Linville, John. "Physician-Assisted Suicide as a Constitutional Right." *Journal of Law, Medicine, and Ethics* 24 (1996): 198–206.

Locke, John. *Second Treatise of Civil Government.* Edited by G. B. Macpherson. Indianapolis: Hackett, 1980.

Mendelssohn, Robert. *Confessions of a Medical Heretic.* Chicago: Contemporary Books, 1979.

Mill, John Stuart. *On Liberty.* In *Utilitarianism, Liberty and Representative Government.* Edited by G. Williams. London: Everyman Library, 1993.

Miller, Franklin, and John Fletcher. "The Case for Legalized Euthanasia." *Perspectives in Biology and Medicine* 36 (1993): 159–76.

Niebuhr, Reinhold. *The Nature and Destiny of Man.* 2 vols. New York: Scribner's, 1941–1943.

Nietzsche, Friedrich. *The Will to Power.* Translated by W. Kaufmann and R. J. Hollingsdale. New York: Vintage Books, 1968.

Novak, David. *Suicide and Morality.* New York: Scholars Studies Press, 1975.

Novum Testamentum Graece. 24th ed. Edited by E. Nestle. Stuttgart: Privileg. Württ. Bibelanstalt, 1960.

Oxford English Dictionary. 2nd ed. 20 vols. Oxford: Oxford University Press, 1989.

Plato. *Apology.* Translated by H. N. Fowler. Cambridge, Mass.: Harvard University Press, 1914.

————. *Crito.* Translated by H. N. Fowler. Cambridge, Mass.: Harvard University Press, 1914.

————. *Euthyphro.* Translated by H. N. Fowler. Cambridge, Mass.: Harvard University Press, 1914.

————. *Laws.* Translated by R.G. Bury. 2 vols. Cambridge, Mass.: Harvard University Press, 1926.

————. *Phaedo.* Translated by H. N. Fowler. Cambridge, Mass.: Harvard University Press, 1914.

————. *Republic.* Translated by P. Shorey. 2 vols. Cambridge, Mass.: Harvard University Press, 1930.

Plutarch. *Plutarch's Lives.* 11 vols. Translated by B. Perrin. Cambridge, Mass.: Harvard University Press, 1959.

Quill, Timothy, et al. "Care of the Hopelessly Ill." *New England Journal of Medicine* 327 (1992): 1380–83.

Ricoeur, Paul. *Oneself as Another.* Translated by K. Blamey. Chicago: University of Chicago Press, 1992.

Seneca. *Epistolae.* 3 vols. Translated by R. W. Gummere. Cambridge, Mass.: Harvard University Press, 1925.

Singer, Peter. *Unsanctifying Human Life.* Edited by H. Kuhse. Oxford: Blackwell, 2002.

Spinoza, Baruch. *Tractatus Theologico-Politicus.* Translated by M. D. Yaffee. Newburyport, Mass.: Focus Publishing, 2004.

Thomas Aquinas. *Summa Theologiae.* In *Basic Writings of Saint Thomas Aquinas.* Translated and edited by A. C. Pegis. 2 vols. New York: Random House, 1945.

Tierney, Brian. *The Idea of Natural Rights.* Atlanta: Scholars Press, 1997.

Warren, Samuel, and Louis Brandeis. "The Right to Privacy." *Harvard Law Review* 4 (1890): 193–220.

Wittgenstein, Ludwig. *Tractatus Logico-Philosophicus.* Translated by D. F. Pears and B. F. McGuinness. London: Routledge and Kegan Paul: 1961.

LEGAL DECISION

Compassion in Dying v. Washington 79 F.3d 790 (9th Cir. 1996). Opinion available at http://caselaw.lp.findlaw.com/scripts/getcase.pl?court =9th&navby=case&no=9435534&exact=1.

INDEX

Note: "Rabbi" or "Rav" in parentheses following a proper name indicates a Talmudic sage.

THE SANCTITY
OF HUMAN LIFE
DAVID NOVAK

In this fascinating study of the theological
and the philosophical, Jewish theologian
David Novak digs deep into Jewish scripture and tradition to find guidance for as-
sessing three contemporary controversies
in medicine and public policy: the use of
embryos to derive stem cells for research,
socialized medicine, and physician-assisted
suicide. Beginning with thinkers like Plato,
Aristotle, Kant, and Nietsche, and drawing
on great Jewish figures in history—Maimonides, Rashi, and various commentators on
the Torah (written law) and the Mishnah
(oral law)—Novak speaks brilliantly to these
modern moral dilemmas.

The Sanctity of Human Life weaves a rich
and sophisticated tapestry of evidence to
conclude that the Jewish understanding of
the human being as sacred, as the image of
God, is in fact compatible with philosophi-